Basic Laboratory Instrumentation for Speech and Hearing

Basic Laboratory Instrumentation for Speech and Hearing

Jack F. Curtis, Ph.D.

Professor, School of Communicative Disorders,
University of Wisconsin/Stevens Point, Stevens Point, Wisconsin

Martin C. Schultz, Ph.D.

Professor, Communication Disorders and Sciences, College of Communications,
Southern Illinois University, Carbondale, Illinois

Little, Brown and Company
Boston/Toronto

Library of Congress Catalog Card No. 85-081752

ISBN 0-316-16552-2

Printed in the United States of America

DON

To Lynn

Contents

Preface

Our goals in this book involve both process and content, medium and message. We see and are trying to meet the need for an introductory book dealing with equipment used in the communicative disorders clinic. We believe that achieving competence in equipment use and mastering the principles underlying such equipment require knowledge of some basic electronics. We have tried to present those basics so that they can be mastered by a reader enrolled in a course or by a reader struggling alone. A representative variety of the types of instrumentation routinely available in the clinic or laboratory is discussed, with emphasis on the principles underlying equipment design.

The message is that you, the reader, can become proficient in choosing and using equipment. Some equipment is technically sophisticated so it is not expected that you will master it instantly. The point is that the conceptual principles are relatively few and simple, certainly far simpler than the client or patient on whose behalf you are using the equipment.

We have tried to keep you in mind in our presentation and in our style. The pathway may be rocky at times but it can be mastered, even at the occasional cost of two steps forward and one step back (one of us remembers it as often being one step forward and two back!). Good luck.

J. F. C.
M. C. S.

Acknowledgments

We feel that this is one of the most pleasurable parts of writing: the chance to acknowledge those who helped along the way. Unfortunately, we cannot acknowledge by name all those students and teachers who have taught us much of what is contained in this book. As we look back, it becomes difficult to decide who was student and who teacher.

Jane Heath Huber encouraged the initial steps and smoothed the way. Her support was boundless and thanks are hardly recompense.

We would also like to thank our colleagues for their help and patience. Dean Burdette Eagon at the University of Wisconsin/Stevens Point assisted by finding funds for typists and artists. Bev Clayton deserves thanks for the clever illustrations that help to convey our ideas in a palatable way. Our typists, Lorraine Bretl and Sharon Donlan, certainly merit gratitude.

James Shapley, a paragon of patience and precision, offered countless wise suggestions that have markedly improved the clarity and accuracy of this book. Without his counsel we would still be struggling.

Introduction

Two Examples

This book is to play two themes, one against the other, with both blending into middle melody. One theme is the variety of clinical and laboratory measures for which one needs equipment; the other is the variety of pieces of equipment that can be used for clinical purposes. The midline includes an introductory understanding of the principles behind instrumentation design, construction, and use, which serves to bridge these complementary themes.

We begin with two commonly occurring situations that are likely to involve our interaction with equipment and, in each, we try to point out what conceptual questions arise and how they are translated into instrumental questions.

EXAMPLE 1

A speech and language pathologist screening transfer students in her school spends some time listening to a boy with a repaired cleft of the palate. She perceives that his voice is not normal, but she is not sure in what way it differs from his classmates' voices. She feels that she needs to hear him again, probably outside the rush of school hours.

She can either request that the boy remain after school and talk until she can make up her mind or she can tape-record a sample of his speech and replay it at her leisure as many times as is necessary to make a decision. She tape-records the boy's speech and on repeated listening determines that the unusual quality may stem from nasal emission. To check her suspicion she visits a nearby university and makes a sound spectrogram. When she finds the visual pattern is similar to those common with nasal emission, she recalls the student to check his nasal emission with a nasal manometer that she has constructed of a glass U tube and a nasal olive.

Let us reconsider some of these steps and their implications. We begin with the clinician hearing some speech and desiring to hear it again, perhaps repeatedly. Her decision is to record some vocal samples; thus she must have control of a microphone, a recording device, a storage medium (the audio tape), and a reproducing device. In addition, (1) the microphone and recording device must be capable of recording the signal faithfully, (2) the audio tape must be capable of storing the sample without distorting it and must be relatively economical, and (3) the reproducing system must be faithful and must not destroy the tape it plays back (in contrast, a camera destroys the film on which it captures any picture by rendering the film unusable for additional pictures).

Our clinician then faced a series of decisions because of her desire to visualize the speech sample. What aspects of the signal should be visualized? What kind of picture would be desirable? How was the tape reproducer to be coupled to the device that would perform the visualization? Finally, she faced an equivalent set of decisions about her validity test of the nasal emission, resulting in the use of a nasal manometer.

How did the clinician even know that one could determine nasal emission from a sound spectrogram? Or, how could the clinician have confidence that her choice of microphone and recorder would capture the strange quality of the boy's speech? She had to make decisions concerning the kind of microphone to use with a tape recorder, the type and quality of recorder, the kind of recording tape, and the kind and quality of reproduction system. Was a sound spectrograph the (most) appropriate device for visualizing nasal emission?

EXAMPLE 2

One day, a therapist in a hospital clinic interviews a man who is suffering vocal strain. The clinician decides that the vocal strain results from habitual use of too low a fundamental pitch, and wants to test her impression. Knowing that good vocal usage is associated with a fundamental pitch approximately one-third of one's total sustainable pitch range, the clinician has her client go on vocal rest for a weekend. He then returns on Monday to record the lowest and highest tones he can sustain and also a sample of his habitual speaking voice. She must now choose some way to extract and measure these three vocal pitches so that, if her impression is correct, she can design a therapy program that might reduce the vocal strain. As we will later discuss, she can choose to use one of at least two general purpose instruments: an oscilloscope or a digital computer; a device of somewhat more limited uses than either of these, a sound spectrograph; or an instrument designed specifically for this purpose, a Visipitch manufactured by Kay Elemetrics.

A general purpose device is widely applicable, but each application requires some set-up and adjustment time. A special purpose device is typically easier to set up and use but then is useful for only that purpose. These advantages and disadvantages must be considered in setting up a laboratory but probably will not concern the ultimate user, the clinician.

We will consider how one analyzes equipment needs and equipment applications, and assist the reader in becoming comfortable with a variety of analysis and display systems. Also, we will consider such issues as decisions about the circumstances under which one chooses a general purpose device or a special purpose device.

In both examples, a clinical problem has been transported into the laboratory to obtain an evaluation that assists therapy. Also, in both cases, the devices that were used were mainly electrical (i.e., not hydraulic or acoustical or mechanical) because electrical devices give us easiest control over the parameters we want to alter or measure. Because most of our instrumentation is electrical, the book has two central foci: the teaching of basic electricity and electronics, and the determination of how devices transfer physical phenomena to or from the electrical domain (e.g., How is air pressure from nasal emission converted into an electrical signal? How is the electrical representation of nasal emission visualized?). This book aims to answer these questions and, more importantly, to teach the clinician how to ask the right questions in order to solve clinical problems.

In the following several chapters, we will consider the various ways a signal can be manipulated. In brief, a signal can be amplified or attenuated, that is, made "bigger" or "smaller" while maintaining its basic fidelity. For this purpose, we will examine amplifiers and volume controls. One particular type of volume control, called an *attenuator*, is calibrated in decibels so as to allow exact control and specification of amplitude change, and we will consider its features among those of other volume controls.

We will examine the principles of *filters*, devices that alter the fidelity of a signal by responding differentially to different frequencies; of *transducers*, devices that change signal energy from one form to another (e.g., light bulb, microphone); of devices that store signals for later use (e.g., tape recorders, computers); and of devices that display signals, measure them, or both. While all transducers change energy from one form to another, some specifically pick up signals (e.g., microphone or physiological electrode), some transducers display signals (e.g., loudspeakers), and we will consider both types in turn. We will also consider principles and practices of evaluating equipment, sometimes to ensure its proper operation, sometimes to consider its relative merit for purchase or for a particular use.

Finally, we will analyze several types of equipment so as to make clear the operational elements of which they are composed. We will also examine several common situations in which the clinician might choose to gain the assistance of instrumentation, in order to analyze what the equipment needs are. Having the reader gain competence in equipment choices and appreciation of her or his own equipment needs is the goal of this book.

I. Basic Principles of
Electricity and Electronics

1. Electricity, Ohm's Law, and Impedance

This first chapter deals with the movement of electrons, which are negatively charged particles. Electron movement is the basis of all electricity, just as some kind of particle movement forms the basis of all phenomena in our world. From time to time, we will show the parallels between electron movement in electricity and movement of other types of particles, such as water molecules flowing in a pipe, to assist in generalizing the principles. But the basis of electricity is particle movement and the work that is done by particles as they move.

Particles move because they have energy. Our conception of the world is based on the idea that the basic source of that energy is (or was) the sun, which provides heat and light energy. The energy from the sun provides heat that is absorbed by particles. That energy is expended in a variety of ways, most especially in random motion (called *Brownian movement*). In this random movement particles release energy, thereby reducing their energy levels. If they all reduced their energy to zero (at 0° Kelvin), there would be no sources of stored energy and all motion would cease. The principle of entropy, a fundamental governing principle of our physical world, states that activity, motion, or energy transfer is in the direction of an even distribution of all energy (and uniform death). In other words, there is a tendency for any pool of energy to be dissipated, for structures (which require energy to be created and for the parts to be brought together and which, thereby, are pools of stored energy) to collapse. As we shall see, electrical activity is the flow of electrons from some pool of stored energy (or from a source creating electrical energy that is fueled by some other pool of energy) toward an even

3

distribution of electrons. But we do have and can create pools of electrical energy, and work can be done in dissipating these pools.

Energy Transfer

In all of the work that we do in our physical world, energy is being used. Often that energy is used by being transferred from one object to another (the energy in the bat is transmitted to the ball it hits) within the same physical domain (the mechanical energy in the bat is transferred to mechanical energy in the ball). Frequently, however, the energy changes form (the acoustical energy in a sound wave is altered to mechanical movement of the eardrum).

A great deal of what we study in speech and hearing involves energy transferring by changing its form (from acoustical to mechanical, hydraulic, or electrical). This process—the change of energy from one form to another or from one domain to another—goes by the formal title of *transduction,* and devices that accomplish the change are *transducers.* A microphone is a transducer that changes acoustical energy to electrical energy; a light bulb is a transducer that changes electrical energy to heat and light energy.

The phenomena we study in speech and hearing arise in any of our physical domains or media: acoustical, hydraulic, mechanical, or electrical, and they frequently appear in more than a single domain. For example, sound (acoustical) impinges on the eardrum, causing it to vibrate (mechanical), which moves the fluid in the inner ear (hydraulic) and thereby moves the basilar membrane (mechanical), triggering neural excitation (electrochemical). The fact that we are called on to deal with phenomena in all four domains requires that we be prepared to use instrumentation in all four domains.

Because the behavior of electronic particles is readily controlled and confined, virtually all instrumentation, for practical purposes, consists of electrical components and of transducers for converting from other media to the electrical and from the electrical back to the other media. Within the electrical or electronic medium, we have devices to alter the amplitude range and to alter the time scale to allow careful examination of phenomena. Our instrumentation accomplishes the tasks we do within the electrical domain.

Simple Harmonic Motion and Waveforms

For purposes of setting the stage of our discussion, we require some common definitions. *Simple harmonic motion* (SHM) can be depicted on a

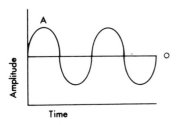

FIG. 1-1. Sinusoidal waveform. A = peak amplitude.

graph, such as a graph describing the displacement of a pendulum from its resting point as a function of time, assuming the pendulum does not gradually stop (SHM is considered to last infinitely long, but a real pendulum will slow down). Graphing the *movement* of a light beam from a flashlight tied to the edge of a wheel moving at constant speed as on a moving car will also result in a pattern of SHM. In the pendulum case, the graph plots the swing of a pendulum over time; in the second, it plots movement of the light through space. In each case we obtain a graph as in Figure 1-1, which displays the magnitude of the swing at each instant in time. The vertical axis, or ordinate, is the magnitude (or amplitude), and the horizontal axis (or abscissa) is time. The graphed wave is sinusoidal because its amplitude varies as the sine of an angle as the angle varies from 0° to 360°. Its magnitude represents the distance of the pendulum from its point of rest or the amplitude of the variation in height of the light as the car wheel revolves and moves. Amplitude A is the peak amplitude. The average amplitude is zero, because the amplitude is symmetrical about zero. Therefore, one may specify peak amplitude but not average amplitude.

COMPLEX WAVEFORMS AND SPECTRA

A sinusoidal waveform may be considered, in some cases, the simplest waveform. Any other repetitive waveform can be broken down into a series of sinusoidal waves of differing amplitudes and repetition rates (i.e., frequencies) and starting locations (phase angles).

Figure 1-2 presents the information in Figure 1-1 in a different form. The repetition rate of the sinusoid is expressed by the frequency (a location on the horizontal axis), and the peak amplitude of the wave is represented by the height of the line. Figure 1-2 is the *line spectrum* of a single sinusoid. Any complex wave that repeats itself (is periodic) can be analyzed into a series of sinusoids, and the series can be displayed as a line spectrum. Figure 1-3 shows the waveform and line spectrum of a

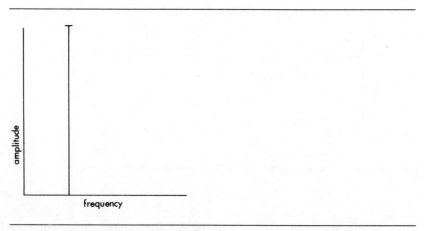

FIG. 1-2.   Line spectrum of a sinusoid.

sawtooth wave. The sawtooth wave consists of a fundamental frequency (f_0) (the rate at which the sawtooth repeats itself) and all the whole-number multiples (called *harmonics* or *overtones*) of that fundamental frequency.

Figure 1-4 displays amplitudes of two sinusoids. The upper curve begins at zero amplitude (i.e., midpoint or rest position in a pendulum swing) and is positive-going (i.e., moving upward). The lower curve begins at the negative-most amplitude and is also positive-going because it is also moving upward. We graph the movement in an up-and-down fashion (+ and −) rather than side-to-side fashion only out of convention.

Why does the upper graph display its curve as starting in positive space (as defined by the ordinate) while the lower graph displays its curve as starting in negative space? The answer lies in the distinction between moving to the left versus being in front of or behind the midpoint of the pendulum swing. Whenever the pendulum is moving forward, it is positive-going, but it is only positive when it is in front of its midpendulum position. This means that the pendulum can be in positive space (in front of its midpoint) whether it is moving to the right or to the left.

The caution for the reader is that *positive* means above the zero line on the graph; *positive-going* means that the curve is moving upward no matter where it is relative to its zero point.

PHASE ANGLE

Simple harmonic motion is graphed as a sinusoid. Phase angle is a measure useful for specifying a point or location on the wave independently of the frequency of the sinusoid. Alternatively, the relation between two

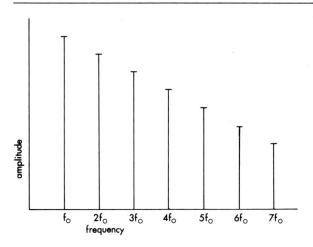

FIG. 1-3. Line spectrum of a sawtooth wave. f_0 = fundamental (lowest) frequency of the wave.

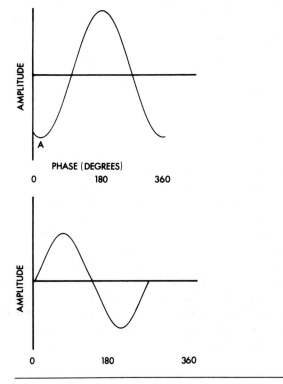

FIG. 1-4. Two sinusoids 90° out of phase.

sinusoids of identical frequency can be stated as a difference in their phase angles. Phase angle derives from simple rotational movement: if one watches a point on the circumference of a wheel moving at a constant rotational velocity, the point shows or undergoes sinusoidal movement.

Because of the derivation of phase angle from circular motion, the measurement of phase angle typically is expressed in degrees from 0° to 360°, with 360° representing one complete cycle of activity from 0°; therefore, both 0° and 360° represent identical locations on the circumference of a circle.

There are two alternative conventions for expressing the location of a point on a sinusoidal wave. In the first, a continuing sinusoid (Fig. 1-4) can be labeled as being at 0° when the curve is at zero amplitude and moving toward positive amplitudes (e.g., the origin of the curve at the top of Fig. 1-4 or the locus of the *A* at the bottom). Alternatively, one can select a point in time and label the graph as 0° (or any other number of degrees) at that point, independently of the amplitude of the wave.

Figure 1-4 displays the convention of labeling both waves from some arbitrary location or point in time. Each wave begins at 0° and shows a complete cycle from 0° to 360°. The bottom wave *lags* the top wave by 90°; that is, any amplitude on the top wave is attained by the bottom wave 90° after it is attained by the top wave. Both waves are sinusoids, are of equal amplitude and frequency, and have a 90° phase relationship (phase angle difference); that is, the top wave *leads* the bottom wave by 90° (or *lags* it by 270° because the top wave is at 270° when it shows the amplitude that is shown by the bottom wave at 0°).

Some Basic Electricity

Most of the equipment we use today is electronic, not mechanical, so that what we actually measure appears as some sort of electrical signal. For instance, if we are measuring airflow from the nose by using an electronic meter, the airflow measure would be displayed as some magnitude of electricity on a meter (even though the meter may be labeled in airflow units). Sometimes the variable we are interested in measuring is actually electrical, as in electromyography, which measures electrical signals associated with muscle activity, but often the energy is not initially in an electrical form. When the variable is not electrical, the electronic measuring device must be able to convert the energy from the form in which it appears, such as air pressure, light, or sound, into electrical energy. Any device that converts energy from one form to another is called a *transducer.*

A good example of a transducer is the phonograph cartridge in a phonograph system. The mechanical energy created by the movement of a stylus in a groove is converted into an electrical signal that is an analogous representation of the wiggle in the record grooves. This analog signal from the cartridge is then amplified and fed to the voice coil of a loudspeaker that converts the electrical energy into acoustical energy by moving the cone of the loudspeaker. Both cartridge and speaker are thus examples of transducers, whereas the amplifier is not a transducer because it does not change energy from one form to another; rather, it only amplifies energy.

Because we deal with electrical signals, we will discuss some of the basic laws of electricity that will be useful. Some of that utility arises because of the intimate relationship that exists among several forms of energy in our world. For example, any hydraulic system can be displayed as an analogous electrical system, acoustical system, or mechanical system. Similarly, any acoustical system can be displayed as a hydraulic, mechanical, or electrical or other system. In addition to the relationship among forms of energy, the relationships that exist within each form can be expressed in mathematical terms so that while each energy system can serve as a model for each of the others, mathematics can also serve as a model for each.

Electrical circuits and components are relatively simple to understand and to master because electrical phenomena are *energic* rather than *synergic.* That is, a circuit can be considered as the sum of its parts (energic) rather than being greater than the sum of its parts (synergic). Even computers, as we shall see, are easy to understand as combinations (often millions of combinations) of relatively few elements and types of simple circuits. Therefore, the mathematics of analyzing most of the kinds of circuits we will require is also simple.

Electricity is a form of energy, and energy is related to motion. The form of motion in electricity is the motion of electrons. Electrons, you likely remember, are those components of an atom that have a negative electrical charge (protons are those elements of an atom that have a positive charge). Atoms typically are electrically neutral because unlike charges attract and each free electron or proton will attract its opposite, if one is available, so that their charges will neutralize, bringing the atom into zero charge.* Therefore, in order to have electrical energy available, one must have a source of electrons that are separated from atoms, which would hold electrons in electrical balance by matching their number with an equal number of protons. In addition, the electrons must have a pathway or pathways through which they can move.

An accumulation of electrons separated from their nuclei is a source

---

*Any discussion of atomic structure is subject to constant revision, especially now with the discovery of new constituent particles within the atom. Our brief discussion here is much simplified but, we hope, sufficient for an understanding of the basis of electricity.

TABLE 1-1.   Common prefixes

Prefix	Abbreviation	Application
Milli– (1/1,000)	m	Usually currents in equipment (e.g., milliampere [mA]) or times in physiological events (milliseconds [ms])
Micro– (1/1,000,000)	μ	Capacitor values (microfarad [μF]) or voltages found in the body (microvolts [μV])
Pico– or micromicro–	p or μμ	Capacitor values
Kilo– (1,000 times)	k	Usually resistor values (kilohms) or frequency (kilohertz [kHz])
Mega–	M	Usually resistor values (megaohms [MΩ])

of potential energy or voltage. The larger the accumulation of charge, the greater the potential to do work because of the work that was done in separating the electrons from their resting atomic states. The measure of charge, the coulomb, represents the magnitude of accumulation of electrons (1 coulomb $= 6.25 \times 10^{18}$ electrons).

MEASUREMENTS

Many of the units of measurement discussed in this book have been derived from industrial applications. The amounts measured are extremely large as compared with the values found in the speech science laboratory. Therefore, a series of prefixes has been devised to denote smaller values. Table 1-1 shows some prefixes for smaller and larger values.

BLOCK DIAGRAMS AND SCHEMATICS

Throughout the book we will be discussing circuits and illustrating them with *block diagrams* or *schematics.* Schematics are more detailed versions of block diagrams. Several symbols that are standard in the professional literature are used in block diagrams and schematics.

In block diagrams, various elements that perform specific functions are illustrated by symbols whose shape or marking identifies them as carrying out the specific functions, but the block diagram does *not* illustrate how the functions are performed. The schematic is much more detailed. It illustrates each of the electronic components in the circuit in sufficient detail that a technician could construct the operating element from the schematic.

This book is not intended to train technicians, so the majority of the illustrations will be in terms of block diagrams. In some cases, schematics will be shown when detail is necessary, as, for example, in Chapter 4,

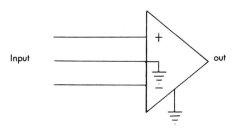

FIG. 1-5.   Block diagram of an amplifier.

where we think it important to show how attenuators and transistors operate.

The block diagram begins with a series of geometric shapes connected by lines. The lines represent wires and cables, and a single line may represent several conductors. The most common block diagram depicts the amplifier, which is shown as a triangle. Usually the flow of signal through a block diagram is from left to right. The amplifier may have two inputs, each with its own hot wire but with a common ground connection (see Ground, following), as shown by Figure 1-5, or more than two inputs.

The + sign at one input denotes that the output is in phase with this input. The − then denotes that the output is 180° out of phase with this input. This means that the output is an amplified version of the input but is inverted so that what is positive at the input is negative at the output and vice versa. Ground, or the common connection between the inputs, is denoted by ⟂ . This symbol is also used in schematics.

Figure 1-6 is a block diagram of a public-address system that demonstrates the use of the symbolic notation common in electronics. Table 1-2 presents many of the commonly used symbols. In some cases, circuit components will be *polarized*. This means that they must be connected in a specific way even though it may look like there is no difference in the component connections. For example, in some circuits, capacitors must be connected with one of the wires at a lower voltage than the other wire. For this reason, many capacitors are labeled with a − or GND (ground) point. On a schematic, the lower voltage or ground connection is represented by a curved line, as shown in Table 1-2.

Some components have only wires coming from unnumbered connections and, if these are not labeled, they may be color-coded. That is, the color of the wire denotes to what it should be connected. This is most often true of transformers, where black wires are usually the ones to be connected to the 110-V input, and the green wires are the "filament" voltages for a vacuum tube circuit, that is, 6 or 12 V. There can be a

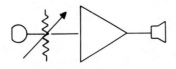

FIG. 1-6.   Block diagram of a public-address system.

multitude of connections, and most electronics manuals list the color codes for transformers and other components.

In order to determine the connections on vacuum tubes, transistors, and integrated circuits, it is necessary to refer to tube manuals and semiconductor manuals available from manufacturers and electronics retailers. Figure 1-7 shows a page from one of the popular semiconductor manuals. Note that the semiconductors are listed in numerical and then alphabetical order. At the top is a brief description of the uses of the integrated circuit (IC), a complete schematic of the circuit contained in the IC, and some sample circuits in which the IC might be used.

GROUND

When connecting devices together in most circuits, one usually finds two wires in the cable, the *hot wire* and the *ground connection*. Two wires are needed because, as has been discussed, there must be two connections to any power source—an outgoing and an incoming line—to establish a complete circuit. A battery, more properly called a *dry cell,* for example, has + and − terminals (Fig. 1-8). The power company that supplies power to a community connects one side of its generators to the earth through a rod driven into the ground—hence the term *ground.* In electrical circuits, one side will be common to most of the elements. This side is designated as the ground. It is called ground because all building wiring is connected at the power company and in your home or office to the earth through a copper rod and also to the white wire (usually) in your wiring system. The other side will be connected in a variety of ways and is labeled as *hot,* because if one were standing on the ground and touched this side of the power line, it would truly be hot (Fig. 1-9).

FUSES AND CIRCUIT BREAKERS

Because too much current can damage equipment or, worse yet, cause a fire, safety precautions related to current flow have been developed. Simply stated, the purpose of a fuse is to prevent too much current from passing through a circuit. All materials have some resistance, with even excellent conductors having a small amount. The resistance comes about because of electrons rubbing against others in passing through a conduc-

TABLE 1-2. Schematic symbols

Symbol	Definition	Note
Resistor	Resistor	
Variable resistor	Variable resistor	
Capacitors	Capacitors	Curved line represents outer plate and is to be connected to lowest voltage point
Variable capacitor	Variable capacitor	For tuning circuits
Inductor	Inductor	Wound on a hollow core or no core
Inductor	Inductor	Wound on a ferrite core
Fuse	Fuse	
Transformer	Transformer	
Push button	Push button	
Relay	Relay	
Switch	Switch (shown in open position so signal cannot pass)	This is an example of one toggle controlling two switches
Transistor	Transistor	
Integrated circuit	Integrated circuit*	There may be as few as 4 or as many as 24 numbered terminals

*An integrated circuit (IC) is a commercial circuit of many different elements that are fabricated into a single unit. An IC is often quite small and may contain hundreds or thousands of circuit elements wired to perform many complex activities, as the magazine ads for Bell Telephone will frequently illustrate.

XR-072

Low-Noise Dual BIFET Operational Amplifier

GENERAL DESCRIPTION

The XR-072 low-noise junction FET input dual operational amplifier is designed to offer higher performance than conventional bipolar dual op-amps. Each of the two op-amps on the chip is closely matched in performance characteristics, and each amplifier features high slew-rate, low input bias and offset currents, and low offset voltage drift with temperature. The XR-072 FET-input dual op-amp is fabricated using ion implanted bipolar/FET or "BIFET" technology which combines well-matched junction FETs and high-performance bipolar transistors on the same monolithic integrated circuit. Its low noise characteristics make it particularly well-suited to low level signal processing, audio preamplification and active filter design.

FEATURES

Direct Replacement for Texas Instruments TL072
High-Impedance Junction FET Input Stage
Internal Frequency Compensation
Low Power Consumption
Wide Common-Mode and Differential Voltage Ranges
Low Input Bias and Offset Currents
Output Short-Circuit Protection
Latch-Up-Free Operation
High Slew-Rate . . . 13V/μs, Typical
Low Noise . . . 18 nV/$\sqrt{Hz}$, Typical

APPLICATIONS

Active Filter Design
Sample/Hold and Servo Systems
Audio Signal Processing
Analog Control Systems

ABSOLUTE MAXIMUM RATINGS

Supply Voltage	±18V
Differential Input Voltage	±30V
Input Voltage Range (Note 1)	±15V
Output Short-Circuit Duration (Note 2)	Indefinite
Package Power Dissipation:	
Plastic Package	625 mW
Derate Above T_A = +25°C	5.0 mV/°C
Ceramic Package	750 mW
Derate Above T_A = +25°C	6.0 mW/°C
Storage Temperature Range	−65°C to +150°C

Note 1: For Supply Voltage less than ±15V, the absolute maximum input voltage is equal to the supply voltage.
Note 2: The output may be shorted to ground or to either supply. Temperature and/or supply voltages must be limited to ensure that the dissipation rating is not exceeded.

AVAILABLE TYPES

Part Number	Package	Operating Temperature
XR-072M	Ceramic	−55°C to +125°C
XR-072N	Ceramic	−25°C to +85°C
XR-072P	Plastic	−25°C to +85°C
XR-072CN	Ceramic	0°C to +75°C
XR-072CP	Plastic	0°C to +75°C

EQUIVALENT SCHEMATIC

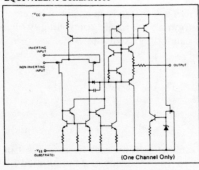

(One Channel Only)

FUNCTIONAL BLOCK DIAGRAM

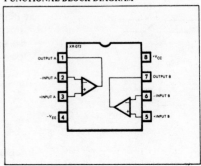

FIG. 1-7.   A page from a semiconductor manual.

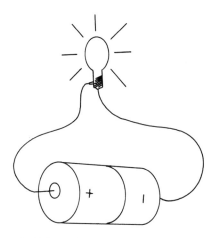

FIG. 1-8.   A simple circuit consisting of a dry cell and a lamp.

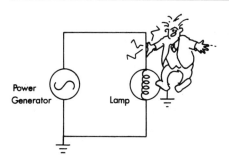

FIG. 1-9.   The possible consequence of touching the "hot" side of the power line.

tor. This rubbing causes the energy that is imparted to the circuit to be converted to heat and light and no longer available to allow the movement of the electrons through the circuit to continue. Obviously, the greater the current that is forced through a conductor, the greater the amount of rubbing that can take place, since there are then many more electrons to rub against one another. If enough rubbing takes place, enough heat will be generated to cause a melting of the conductor, causing a complete change of the state of the material. This is the principle of the fuse. A fuse consists of a small piece of wire through which the current must pass. The diameter of the wire determines the amount of current that can pass through it before it will melt. To protect a circuit it is a simple matter to put a fuse in the circuit that will melt if more than

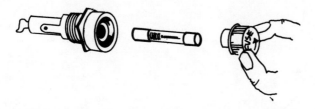

FIG. 1-10.   A fuse and fuse holder of the type commonly found in electronic instruments.

the needed current flows through it. Since the fuse is part of the circuit, the melting of the wire causes the circuit to become open and discontinuous so that no more current can flow. Figure 1-10 shows a fuse of the type commonly found in electronic equipment in the speech clinic. The value of the fuse (the amount of current that can flow before the fuse melts) is stamped on the metal ends of the fuse.

In many devices there is a large surge of current when the equipment is first turned on because of the charging of the capacitors in the power supply, but this initial surge is quickly followed by a much smaller constant current during normal operation. If a standard fuse were used, the initial surge, which is perfectly normal, would cause the fuse to melt, or "blow." To overcome this initial surge problem, slow-blow fuses have been developed. These are simply fuses that allow a large amount of current to flow for a moment, but then the amount must decrease to the value stated on the fuse or the fuse will blow. Slow-blow fuses should never be used to replace the standard type of fuse in other kinds of devices since damage to the equipment could result if a momentary surge occurred where it should not. It is all right to use normal fuses in place of slow-blow fuses, but such fuses will often blow when you try to operate the equipment (even though the equipment is operating properly) because they are designed to have an initial surge.

Circuit breakers were developed to eliminate the trouble and expense of replacing fuses. Circuit breakers are devices that consist of switches that can be latched on and held in position by a piece of springy metal through which the current in the circuit will flow. As current flows through the spring, it causes the spring to change shape and, when the shape is changed sufficiently, the switch opens. The relationship between the release of the spring and the current through it can be precisely controlled, so it is possible to construct circuit breakers that control specified amounts of current. Once the breaker is triggered, the reason for the excess current is corrected and then the breaker is latched again. Many modern circuits, especially integrated circuits, cannot use circuit breakers because the circuit elements can burn up before the breaker

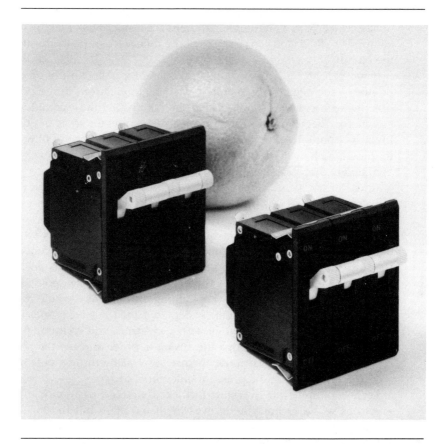

FIG. 1-11.   Circuit breakers used in laboratory equipment and microcomputers. (Courtesy Heinemann Electric Co., Lawrenceville, NJ.)

opens. As a matter of fact, a great deal of research was necessary to develop fuses that would blow before the circuits. Figure 1-11 illustrates a circuit breaker of the type commonly found on a digital computer.

A SIMPLE DIRECT CURRENT CIRCUIT

The principles behind electrical circuits are conceptually simple. They arise from the very fundamental tendency of nature to equalize physical differences (water seeks a common level; hot objects cool to the temperature around them or cold ones heat up; living bodies die and decay to revert to the elements constituting them)—the principle of entropy. This principle implies that electrons will flow only if there is some path (a circuit) and if there is an uneven distribution of electrons in the circuit. That is, the first requirement for current flow is a pool of "excess" electrons, which we call a *voltage source*. Second, the voltage source must connect into a circuit so that there is a route (a complete path) for electrons to flow along so as to distribute themselves equally throughout the circuit.

If we consider a battery, which consists of a collection of electrons pooled at the negative pole and an absence of electrons at the positive pole, we can create a simple circuit by connecting the two poles by a conductor. Electrons will flow through the conductor so as to equalize their distribution in the circuit. Eventually, they will cease to flow, since there will no longer be any pressure differential (and the battery will be completely discharged and "dead").

Consider the same, initially charged battery, and now connect its terminals to the leads of a light bulb. Again, electrons will attempt to flow, but their path is now through the light bulb. The bulb uses as a conductor a wire that impedes electron flow, causing the electrons to "rub" together, generating heat that makes the wire blow, thereby converting the flow into light energy and heat energy. The electrons cannot easily flow from the negative pole of the battery to the positive pole as they are converted to doing the work of lighting the bulb. As the bulb remains lit the pool of electrons is gradually depleted and the battery runs down. Until the battery is exhausted, however, electrons will continue to flow from the negative pole through the circuit in order to reach the positive pole, and in order to distribute themselves equally throughout the circuit, thereby bringing the pressure differential to zero.

Let us continue our overview further. If a circuit has multiple paths, electrons will distribute themselves in all the paths but they will flow more easily through the paths where the flow is easier. That is, if we were to establish two paths between our + and − battery terminals, one path consisting of a piece of wire and the other consisting of a light bulb (see Fig. 1-8), some very few electrons would flow through the bulb's "leg" of the circuit, but most would flow through the plain wire because the wire path is easier (the plain wire impedes the electron flow a minute amount so some electrons will go through the bulb; if the plain wire offered no resistance at all then no electrons would flow through the bulb).

It is customary to speak of electrons flowing for the purpose of doing work, such as lighting a bulb, rather than flowing to equalize the electrical pressure, and that custom will be followed in this work. But the reader may be assisted in understanding circuits and circuit elements by remembering the principle of entropy—if there is a circuit and some potential difference, then electrons must flow until the potential difference drops to zero and there is the same potential at all paths, with proportionally more flowing in paths that offer proportionally less resistance to their flow.

Resistance and Ohm's Law

The composition of a conductor will determine the amount of opposition to electrons moving through it. The situation is analogous to moving a heavy block of stone over a rough floor. Because of the unevenness, some of the force applied to the stone is wasted in friction as the block scrapes along the floor. This friction creates heat, thereby converting some of the mechanical energy to thermal energy. In the electrical system, if the wire offers a great deal of resistance, the electrons will rub against one another and create heat, which is, in this case, wasted energy. The electrical friction, called *resistance,* is equivalent to the mechanical friction. If the floor and block were polished, the block could move more easily. It will not make any difference how fast or in what direction the block of stone is pushed. The rough floor will result in wasted effort regardless of anything other than the condition of the opposing surfaces. In electrical terms, this means that the amount of resistance, which is measured in the unit ohm (Ω), is a function of the conductor and is constant regardless of the frequency of the signal and the voltage. Resistors in electronic circuits are typically manufactured from carbon compounds and various types of resistive wires.

Figure 1-12 shows several types of resistors. The physical size of the resistor is a function of the power (power, defined later, relates to the rate at which work can be performed) the resistor is designated to handle. As there is, by convention, a color coding system for marking resistances, the resistance of a given resistor can be determined from the colored bands on the body.

The magnitudes of the source voltage and the resistance determine the amount of electron flow through the circuit; no more can flow through than the amount necessitated by the work done in overcoming the resistances. The basic relationship, called *Ohm's law,* is that the flow of electrons, called the *current,* is the product of the source voltage, which is the push or force acting on the electrons, divided by the resistance:

$$\frac{\text{Voltage}}{\text{Resistance}} = \text{Current}$$

The electromagnetic force, or voltage, is abbreviated as EMF (or E), the resistance is abbreviated R, and the current as I, so that Ohm's law is also stated as E/R = I.

In assessing speech behavior, we deal with energy in many forms. Up until now, we have been talking about electrical energy flow; let us consider a water flow system as an analogy. We will find that the behavior of the circuit elements is identical in both systems.

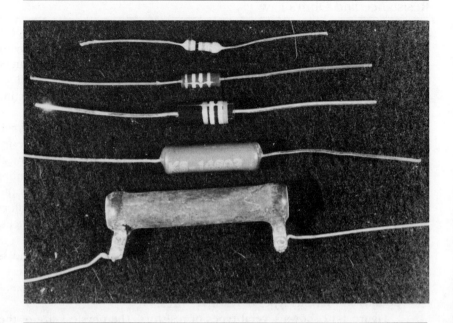

FIG. 1-12.   Resistors of various sizes (wattage ratings). The largest is 54 mm long.

When water flows in a hydraulic system, a specific number of water molecules flow past a given point in a unit of time. This is the *flow rate*, which is analogous to *current*. By *flow rate* in an electrical circuit we mean the number of electrons per unit of time. Remember, however, that since all electrons always travel at the same speed (the speed of light), an increase of flow rate means *more* electrons, not *faster* electrons. (It is important to bear in mind that the flow rate does not specify the total amount of water nor does it tell us anything about the work that the water can do as it moves.)

Water pressure, which is analogous to *voltage,* from a pump or a storage tank moves the water from a point of high pressure to a point of lower pressure. If the pipe is small, there will be great resistance and less water will flow. We can think about water flowing from a particular location through a series of pipes and passing by a series of outlets, with the last outlet releasing the final portion of the expended fluid at some remote location, where the fluid enters the earth to be pumped out again to complete the circuit. When current flows, the amount of current is inversely related to the resistance in the circuit—the smaller the opposition to flow, the greater the flow (i.e., the lower the resistance, the higher the current).

To make the analogy between the hydraulic system discussed above and an electrical system, consider a battery and a wire connecting the poles of the battery. The battery is a source of electrical pressure.* Voltage is equivalent to the quantity of electrons stored in a given unit of area. Current is the quantity of electrons that do flow, and is determined by the relationship between available energy (EMF) and ease of transmission, where the transmission is easier with low resistance (big pipes and faucets) and more difficult with higher resistance (smaller pipes and faucets).

Current flows in the wire. Current is measured in amperes (A) and represents the number of electrons flowing per unit of time past a fixed point. If the wire is large and made of material that is a good conductor, it has a low resistance, and a large current flows. If the resistance increases, less current flows. Resistance varies with the type of material and the diameter of the wire. The greater the voltage, the more current will flow in a wire of some fixed resistance; the lower the resistance, the more current will flow for some fixed voltage.

Early scientists hypothesized that there was a flow in the wire akin to a fluid, and the movement was often described in terms of a liquid. Later, when the interior of the atom was explored, it was discovered that the flow consisted of the movement of electrons, which, as already noted, are negatively charged particles. The movement was from a point of relative excess of electrons ($-$) to a point of relative lack of electrons ($+$).

Consider the circuit in Figure 1-13 and see what will happen. We have connected a 10-V battery to a 10-Ω resistor. Using Ohm's law, we find:

$$E/R = I$$
$$10/10 = I$$
$$= 1 \text{ A}$$

If we now connect several resistors to the battery we have a series circuit. Figure 1-14 shows a series circuit consisting of three resistors and a battery.

To return to the electrical circuit, the amount of current flowing is the same at any point in the series circuit. Therefore, resistance may best be thought of as the friction in the pipe through which the water flows. That is, each element in a water system uses some amount of water pressure

---

*A battery usually consists of two plates of dissimilar materials and an electrolyte in liquid or paste form. If the electrolyte is liquid, the battery is called a *wet cell* (an automobile battery is a wet cell battery). If it is paste, the battery is called a *dry cell* (e.g., a flashlight battery). What we commonly call a battery may be only one cell, which is one positive plate and one negative plate. Automobile batteries have several cells, usually wet.

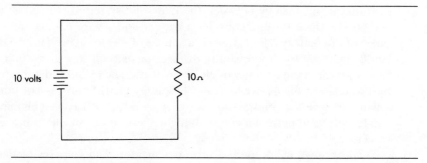

FIG. 1-13.   Simple DC circuit.

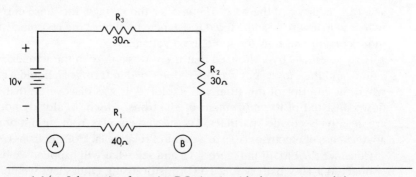

FIG. 1-14.   Schematic of a series DC circuit with three resistors (R).

to push the water through it. Each element having resistance can be thought of as a location reducing some of the pressure through it—the smaller the pipe, the higher the resistance.

Each element of an electrical circuit requires energy (electrons) to work; each resistance uses up (leaks out as heat) electrons. The higher the resistance, the greater the energy used in moving electrons. To continue the analogy, resistors may be used in conjunction with other elements to control the energy that flows to the other elements of the circuit. Sometimes a resistor serves a very different function, as when the resistance of the filament of a light bulb causes it to glow, or causes a heater wire to warm air or water when the resistance uses electrons in the form of heat.

In contrast to the current, the voltage drop varies among different points in the series circuit, as in Figure 1-14. In order to push the electrons through one resistor, a portion of the available EMF will be expended. The pressure differential that remains is used to push the electrons through the other resistors. Thus, part of the EMF is used in each resistor. Therefore, total EMF $(E_t) = E_1 + E_2 + E_3$. Or, if there are more than two resistors, the total equals the sum of all the parts. The result of this principle is that there are different amounts of EMF present at various points relative to ground in the circuit. In a series circuit, the voltage varies across each resistor, but the sum of amounts used in each of the elements must equal the total available.

Resistance is the third element in Ohm's law. In a series circuit in which resistors are strung together, the total resistance (R_t) equals the sum of the resistances in the circuit. The equation is written: $R = R_1 + R_2$, or, if there are more than two: $R = R_1 + R_2 + \ldots + R_n$. Recalling the water analogy, the amount of water that can flow in any part of the system must be the same, but cannot be more than is allowed by the total opposition offered by all the pipes. If there is one small pipe and all the others are large, no more water can flow in any of the larger pipes than can flow through the smallest. In aerodynamic terms, as in the vocal tract, the amount of air that is allowed to flow per unit of time, called the *volume velocity* (analogous to electrical current), is determined by the alveolar pressure and by the sum of the resistances offered by any constriction in the vocal tract.

To continue with the acoustical analogy, consider the case in which the velopharyngeal mechanism is at rest and alveolar pressure is increased. Air flows from the lungs to the oropharynx, and at this point can travel either through the oral cavity or through the nasal cavity. There are two paths, each with a specific amount of resistance.

Figure 1-15 is an electrical analog of the acoustical system just described. The resistors are side by side, that is, in parallel, and the circuit is called a *parallel circuit*. Electrons move from the − pole. Some pass through the 100-Ω resistor and some through the 200-Ω resistor. The EMF is the same at both resistors, but different amounts of current flow through each resistor because of the different resistances to the flow.

Applying the water analogy to the circuit: the source of water pressure, either a pumping station or a water tower, applies the same pressure to each faucet in the home. The amount of water that can flow from the faucet is a function of the diameter of the pipe, so although the flow can vary, the water pressure is constant at each point. In a parallel circuit, the total current (I_t) is the sum of the currents through each element. The equation is: $I = I_1 + I_2 + \ldots + I_n$. Because the current (or the water) has a choice of directions, the total opposition to flow is less than any one of the resistances (R). The equation for total resistance is: $1/R_t = 1/R_1 + 1/R_2 + \ldots + 1/R_n$.

Applying the above principles to the circuit in Figure 1-13, the current can be determined with Ohm's law.

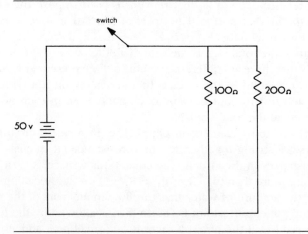

FIG. 1-15.   A parallel DC resistor circuit.

$$\frac{1}{R_t} = \frac{1}{R_1} + \frac{1}{R_2} \qquad\qquad I_t = \frac{50}{66.67} \qquad\qquad I_{R_1} = \frac{E}{R_1} = \frac{50}{100} = 0.5 \text{ A}$$

$$= \frac{1}{100} + \frac{1}{200} \qquad\qquad I_t = 0.75 \qquad\qquad I_{R_2} = \frac{E}{R_2} = \frac{50}{200} = 0.25 \text{ A}$$

$$R_t = 66.67 \qquad\qquad\qquad\qquad\qquad\qquad I_t = I_{R_1} + I_{R_2}$$

$$= 0.5 + 0.25$$

$$= 0.75 \text{ A}$$

Notice that the total current is greater than that which could flow through either resistor alone.

Electronic circuits can become quite complicated, given the possibilities of having a variety of elements in series and in parallel. The issues that concern us in this work do not involve us in the details of circuit construction or circuit analysis; our desire is to gain some appreciation of equipment and its use, more at a component level than at a circuit level. The general principles of circuit analysis are few, however, and an overview can be easily mastered. The two simple principles governing series and parallel circuits are:

A. *The algebraic sum of the sources of voltage and the voltage drops in any complete (or closed) circuit must be zero.*
B. *The current flowing onto any junction must be equal to the current*

leaving that junction (it cannot divide or recombine into a larger or smaller amount).

Using just these two principles and some additional principles we already know, we can derive some conceptual steps that allow complex circuit analysis.

1. In any series circuit, the same current flows through every element; the voltage drop through each element will vary directly with its resistance ($E = IR$, therefore, $I = E/R$; if I is constant, as R increases, E increases).

2. In any parallel circuit, there is the same voltage drop in each parallel arm. Therefore, if the resistances differ from parallel arm to parallel arm, the currents in each parallel arm will also differ so that the voltage drop remains identical. Because the current has multiple paths, more current will flow through the parallel circuit than will flow in any single parallel arm.

3. Circuit analysis always proceeds by considering parallel portions first, and substituting series circuit portions for them. Any parallel circuitry can, for analysis purposes, have a series circuit substituted for it. The series substitution must result in the same voltage drop as occurs across the entire parallel circuit.

4. The circuit analysis in any complex series-parallel circuit proceeds by a progressive substitution of series elements for parallel branches until the entire circuit is represented by a single series circuit.

To return to the acoustical analogy, consider the case of the velopharyngeal port in the vocal tract. When it is completely closed, the electrical analog would be a series circuit through the oral cavity alone, as previously considered. Any opening of the port creates a parallel circuit, and the amount of airflow through the oral and nasal passages is determined by the relative openness of each. The air pressure in each passageway is the same since the voltage drop is identical across parallel arms of an electrical circuit.

In the operation of most equipment, the amount of work performed is the most important consideration. In washing an automobile, for example, if the water pressure is high but there is very little water, it is difficult to move much dirt. Conversely, if there is a great deal of water, but little pressure, the result is the same. The amount of work that can be performed is a function of both the pressure and the amount of water. In electrical circuits, *work*, or *power*, is the result of both electrical pressure (voltage) and current flow. Power is equal to the EMF times the I ($P = E \times I$), and the units are *watts* (W). The product, watts, expresses potential for performing work, and watts multiplied by time gives the rate at which the work is done and, therefore, the rate at which energy is used.

In performing any sort of work, a system will use energy. Energy is used when sound travels into the ear, and the body burns energy while breathing or speaking. Energy varies with the total amount of work performed and is equal to the rate at which energy is expended times the duration of the work. Thus, energy equals power times time. The reader may have noted that electric bills are based on kilowatt hours used: thousands of watts for a given number of hours. This is because the user pays for the electricity consumed in doing work, and is charged for the power consumed for the period in which it is being used.

Electricity and Magnetism

All electrical phenomena occur because some potential difference finds a circuit through which to discharge its excess electrons. Electrons flow toward locations having fewer electrons (i.e., locations having less negative charge or more positive charge). So far, sources of potential difference have been considered that result in electron flow in a single direction only, because the source has some constant value of voltage that is only in one direction. It is much more common in our world to find and use voltage sources that are variable in electron flow. Not only do they vary in value, but the flow is first in one direction in a circuit, then reverses to flow in the opposite direction, then reverses again, many times per second. Continually reversing sources produce *alternating current* (AC) as opposed to electron flow in a single direction (called *direct current,* or DC).

Again, the principles are not difficult, and an overview of them follows. The principles arise because of the intimate linkages of electrical and magnetic phenomena, so that an understanding of AC will arise from a review of the properties of magnets and magnetism. Any magnet exhibits properties of attraction and repulsion for other magnetic material. The magnet has lines of force that surround it. In a bar magnet, these lines of force radiate from one pole to the other. If any material capable of being magnetized enters the field of these lines of force, the material will be magnetized by the field so that it may become a magnet itself. The magnetic polarization of this secondary material will be so induced that the end of the newly magnetized material nearer to the north magnetic pole of the primary magnet will be polarized as a south pole (opposites attract). The greater the magnetic properties of a material and the more massive the material, the stronger a magnet it can become; the closer together the two poles of a magnet, the greater will be the concentration of the radiated lines of force between them.

A horseshoe-shaped magnet will have highly concentrated lines of force because its two ends are close together. If we were to move a copper wire through its force field, the wire would become polarized, with some of its excess electrons moving to one end, leaving an excess of protons at the other. Move it further into the field and the wire becomes more polarized, that is, more electrons move to the one end, leaving more protons at the other. Turn the wire over, thereby reversing it in the force field, and the electron and proton pools must reverse locations. Keep the wire still but reverse the magnet so that the poles now occupy opposite places from before, and again the electrons must flow to the opposite end of the wire. Thus, moving a wire in a magnetic field can cause a current to flow in a wire without any other source of EMF. It is also true that if a current is flowing in a wire and this wire is placed close to another it can cause a current to flow in the second wire, just as if a source of EMF were connected.

Note what has been said: merely by moving a wire through the force field of a magnet, electrons are caused to flow. Moving either the wire or the magnet results in an induced current flow. Further, if electrons flow in one direction while the wire is being moved *into* the field, they will flow in the opposite direction while it moves *out of* the field; that is, reversing direction of the movement of wire relative to the magnet reverses the direction of current flow in the wire.

These basics make an understanding of voltage generators quite simple. A generator, conceptually, is a loop of wire that is rotated within the force field of a magnet. As one side of the wire loop moves toward the positive pole, electrons will move in one direction in the wire; as the wire passes closest to the + pole and begins to move away from it, the direction of electron flow reverses. The direction of flow reverses again as the wire passes closest to the − pole and begins again to move toward the + pole. If a loop of wire is rotated in a magnetic field and the induced current flow is fed to the power line, it provides the alternating current that is available for any use at any outlet. If the loop rotates at some constant rate, then the output AC voltage is sinusoidally shaped, with a frequency that is the rotation rate. Generators in the United States rotate 60 times per second, so house current is 60 Hz AC; many European countries and Canada use 50 Hz AC.

For most circuits in equipment of interest to us, the circuit voltages are those of the signal, not those powering the device, and so the frequencies with which we will be concerned are those making up the frequency composition of the signal. By contrast, whatever voltages must be supplied to ensure the equipment operates will likely enter it as 60 Hz AC, but they will be changed to DC by the power supply and reduced to whatever values are required for the individual circuit elements. To return to the major point, when we discuss frequency content and frequency-sensitive elements, we are referring to signal frequency, not to the house current frequency. The way current flows in a circuit and the functions that a circuit performs can be very different from simple DC circuits when signal voltages vary in frequency and when the circuit contains components that respond differentially to different frequencies.

Impedance

Opposition to energy flow in alternating current circuits is called *impedance* (Z), which consists of two components: *resistance* (R) and *reactance* (X). Reactance varies with the frequency of the signal while resistance, which is constant, does not. The equation is:

$$Z = \sqrt{R^2 + X^2}$$

When electrical circuits include elements that are frequency-sensitive (where the value of the element in the circuit is related to the frequency of the alternating current in the circuit), they require somewhat more complex mathematics. Where the current or flow in the circuit is direct current (f = 0 Hz), then the values of the frequency-sensitive elements are also non-varying, and the mathematics is likewise reduced in complexity.

Reactive elements are of two general types: *inductances* have a small reactance (small opposition to flow) to currents of low frequency and, as the frequency rises, the inductive reactance (opposition to flow) increases; *capacitances* have a large reactance to currents of low frequency and, as the frequency rises, the capacitive reactance decreases. That is, inductances pass most energy (have low impedance and high admittance) for low frequencies; capacitances pass most energy for high frequencies.

One can think about the transfer of electrical energy through a circuit having reactive elements by measuring the impedance, or by considering the reciprocal quantity, the ease of energy transfer, called *admittance.*

Current flow in circuits with reactive elements is complicated by the fact that the currents going through capacitive elements are not in phase with the currents going through inductive elements, and neither is in phase with the currents traveling through resistive elements.

An understanding of the magnitude of the current flow in a circuit as a result of some mixture of differing elements (resistive and reactive) can be furthered if we digress to consider the concept of *vector quantities* and how a vector is calculated. Initially let us consider a simple example. If a sailboat is being pushed by a motor toward a point due

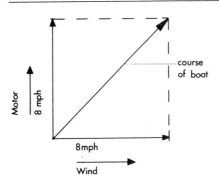

FIG. 1-16.   Vectors applied to seamanship.

north at a speed of 8 miles per hour and is being pushed by the wind toward a point due east at 8 miles per hour, the uncorrected course of the boat would be northeast. The force on the boat in the northerly direction and the force in the easterly direction are of equal magnitude, so that the boat moves in a direction controlled by the equal contribution of both. We could graph this event as seen in Fig. 1-16. In the figure, two forces are represented as operating on the boat. Each has a magnitude and each has a direction; therefore, each is a vector quantity. The resultant vector force is derived from taking into account the relative magnitudes and their directions of action.

The boat is being pushed upon by 8 units of force from the motor, so the magnitude can be graphed as a line 8 units long in that direction. In like manner, the wind is pushing due east on the boat with 8 units of force, which can also be graphed as a line 8 units long in its proper direction. These two forces are graphed as two legs of a triangle, and the resultant vector force is the hypotenuse of the triangle. If the graph were drawn to scale, the actual resultant could be obtained as a measure of the hypotenuse itself on the graph.

A vector quantity, therefore, has both a magnitude and a direction. For example, *velocity* (defined as some speed in some direction) is a vector quantity, whereas speed alone is not. Because vector quantities include the direction in which the action is being effected, it is easy to determine a vector resultant of simple forces by doing a proportional plotting of each force on graph paper and constructing the triangle with its legs representing any two vector forces and the hypotenuse then representing the resultant force of their combination.

INDUCTANCE

When current flows through a wire, magnetic lines of force exist around the wire in much the same way that a magnet has lines of force around

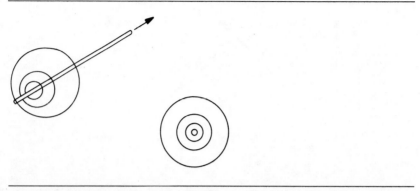

<small>FIG.</small> 1-17.   Magnetic lines of force around a conductor when current is flowing.

it. These lines of force may be visualized as concentric circles around the conductor, as in Figure 1-17. If the current is large, there are many lines of force and they radiate quite a distance from the wire. If the current is small, there are few lines and they are close to the wire. The number of lines of force determines the *field strength*. As current begins to flow in a conductor, a magnetic field builds around it to a strength determined by the composition of the conductor and the magnitude of the current. If the current is steady, the field stabilizes at this strength (and does so quite rapidly) so long as the steady current flows. If the current increases, the field expands; if current decreases, the field strength shrinks. When the current is turned off, the field collapses. Once a steady current begins to flow, the magnetic lines of force are fixed around the wire and are stable. That is, when current flows through a wire, the wire resembles a magnet, with comparable attraction and repulsion characteristics.

If the wire is coiled, the lines of force tend to assume a shape around the coil as shown in Figure 1-18. In addition, one end of the coil becomes a north pole and the other a south pole (defined by their relative attraction or repulsion to the earth's polarity), just as in a permanent magnet. That is, the south pole of a magnet is attracted to the North Pole of the earth. If the coil is formed around a piece of soft iron, an electromagnet is formed.

Inductance (L) is a property of magnetic lines of force; it is determined by the physical parameters of the coil, such as diameter, size of the wire, and number of turns, and is expressed in henrys. When a conductor cuts magnetic lines of force, a current is *induced* in that conductor. The word *cut* as used here means that a conductor is passed through the magnetic lines of force or vice versa. In Figure 1-19A, a wire is connected to a battery. In Figure 1-19B, a wire is connected to a meter but with no physical connection to part A. If either part is moved closer to the other,

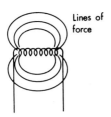

FIG. 1-18. Lines of force around a coil.

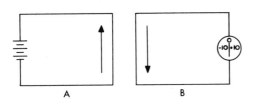

FIG. 1-19. Circuit illustrating the property of inductance. See text for details.

the meter will deflect during the movement, showing that a current is flowing. It is important to remember that the lines must move *through* the wire or the wire must move *through* the lines, or both. If the lines are stable and the wire is stable, nothing will happen. This is demonstrated by the circuit in Figure 1-19. If A and B move closer together the meter will deflect toward − 10. If they are moved apart the meter will deflect toward + 10. Once the movement ceases, the meter will return to zero.

The current induced in part B flows in the opposite direction from the field of magnetic lines of force flowing in part A. This is shown by the arrows in Figure 1-19. If the wires are moved away from one another, the current flows in the same direction in both parts during that movement. Because any conductor with current flowing through it is surrounded by a field of magnetic lines of force, physically moving an element back and forth in a DC circuit has the same effect on elements of nearby circuits as would the expanding and collapsing fields of a varying AC current. The general rule is: A conductor coming into a magnetic field has a current induced in it in a direction opposite to that of the field (the attraction of opposites). A conductor moving out of a magnetic field has a current induced in it in the same direction as the field.

Figure 1-20 shows a battery connected to a wire as in Figure 1-19, but

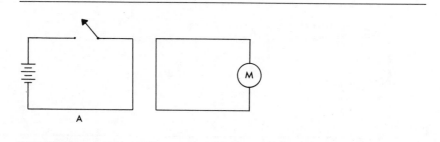

FIG. 1-20.   Circuit of Figure 1-19 with added switch. M = meter.

a switch has been added. When the switch is open, as shown, there is no current flow and thus no magnetic lines of force. If the switch is closed, current begins to flow and the magnetic lines of force begin to radiate out from the wire-like rings on the surface of a pond when a stone is thrown into it. These lines cut the second conductor and a current is induced in the opposite direction from the primary current. However, after the switch has been closed long enough for the field to be created, the lines stabilize and reach maximum strength and no longer move. *There is no induced current once stability is achieved.*

From this discussion, it is apparent that a current may be induced by the conductor moving through the lines of force or by the *lines of force moving through the conductor.* Anything causing a change in the relationship between the second conductor and the lines of force will result in an induced current.

If the switch is opened, the lines of force collapse and squeeze back into the conductor. During this collapse, the lines cut the secondary conductor in the opposite direction, and current flows in the same direction that the primary current, *when it was flowing,* followed.

In DC circuits, the push is in one direction and is usually constant, but in AC circuits the push varies. The EMF continuously changes in magnitude and direction over time. What happens to magnetic fields when this kind of alternating voltage is applied to a wire? Magnetic lines of force radiate out, collapse, and radiate out again. When the lines that gradually expand cut the second conductor, they induce a current flow in the opposite direction from the original current. When the initial current flow is interrupted, the lines of force begin to collapse. This time the lines are cutting the second conductor in the opposite direction; that is, instead of cutting as in Figure 1-21A, they are cutting as in Figure 1-21B. This time the induced current is in the same direction as the original current.

If the direction of primary current flow is changed, the induced current also changes direction and is then going in the opposite direction

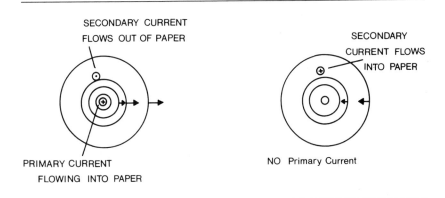

SECONDARY CURRENT
FLOWS OUT OF PAPER

SECONDARY
CURRENT FLOWS
INTO PAPER

PRIMARY CURRENT
FLOWING INTO PAPER

NO Primary Current

FIG. 1-21.   Induced current when lines of force are expanding (A) and
collapsing (B).

from the primary (this induced current flow is now in the same direction
as the initial one).

When an EMF begins to push a current through a wire, magnetic lines
of force are set up around the wire and cut any neighboring conductors,
inducing a current in the opposite direction when they are expanding,
and in the same direction when they are collapsing. In a coil of wire, the
turns of the coil lie side by side and each turn is essentially a conductor
lying next to a conductor. If a current flows through the wire, the lines
of force cut the neighboring conductor. It makes no difference to the
wire or the lines of force that the conductor is also part of the primary
conductor—*current is still induced in the opposite direction.* This
means that a source of voltage is pushing electrons in one direction, and
induced current is flowing in the opposite, as if you had connected a
source of voltage opposite to the real one. This property is called *back
EMF.* Back EMF tends to reduce the flow of current because the source
is pushing in one direction and the back EMF is pushing in the opposite
direction. In the case of a constant direction current, once the forward
push stabilizes and the lines of force become stable, current can flow
normally. Then, if the magnitude or direction changes, the lines again
induce a back EMF. This means that if the EMF is varying as a sinusoid,
the current will also be a sinusoid, but *not in phase* (because of this
difference in direction). Figure 1-22 shows the voltage and the current
in a circuit consisting of a source and a coil. In a purely inductive circuit,
the current is 90° behind the voltage. The current is doing what the
voltage "wanted it to do" 90° ago. Thus, with a sinusoidal wave in which
the push is varying in magnitude and direction as a sinusoid, the induced

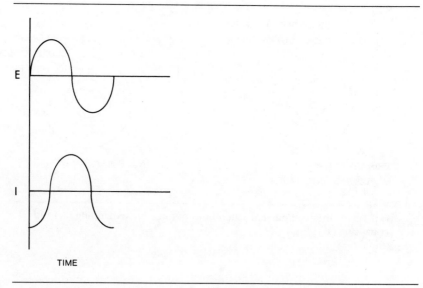

FIG. 1-22.   Voltage (E) and current (I) relationships in an inductor.

current varies as a sinusoidal wave, but not in step with the primary current.

Inductive reactance, the opposition to flow in an inductor, provides a very useful analog to *mass* in a mechanical system. Newton stated that a mass at rest tends to remain at rest until acted on by an outside force. *Inertia* is the name given to this tendency for mass to continue without change whatever state it is in. When a force is applied to a mass, the inertia of the mass must be overcome in getting it to move. It takes much more energy to start a car rolling on a flat road than it does to keep it moving since the car's inertia opposes any change. Thus the car requires more energy to start it rolling than to keep it rolling. The situation is analogous to a coil to which an electromotive force is applied. The current does not begin to flow until the magnetic lines of force stabilize and the back EMF is reduced.

Newton also said that a body in constant motion tends to remain in constant motion until acted on by an outside force. In the coil, the current flows until back EMF is again introduced into the current. That is, once a current is flowing, any change in the current, either increasing or decreasing it, will induce an opposing back EMF.

RESISTOR-INDUCTOR COMBINATIONS

Figure 1-23, a graph of the voltage and current relationship in a resistor over time, illustrates this discussion. Resistance is the analog of friction,

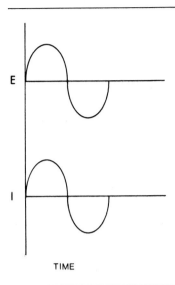

FIG. 1-23.   Voltage (E) and current (I) relationships in a resistor.

and friction is present regardless of the direction and magnitude of the EMF. Current and EMF are in phase in a resistance.

If an alternating source of EMF, or AC, is connected to a resistor and a coil, each influences current flow (i.e., instantaneous currrent amplitude) according to its own characteristics. The resultant current flow in the circuit will be a joint product of the relative influence of each. Let us consider the influences individually and then combine them. Because the total current is the sum of the currents at each instant in time, if the current is graphed, the resultant will be the sum through the resistor plus the sum through the coil at each instant in time. Consider a series circuit containing both a resistor and a coil as in Figure 1-24. What is the current relationship in the circuit? The current in the resistor will be in phase with the source (and with the voltage) for the resistor alone, and that in the coil will be 90° out of phase (delayed relative both to the source and to the resistor) for the coil alone. The resultant current for the combination will be determined by the addition of the current in the resistor alone and the current in the coil alone at each instant in time.

If the opposition to current flow in the coil (reactance) is equal to the opposition to current flow in the resistor (resistance), the current will be 45° out of phase. Figure 1-25 illustrates the resultant for equal current in each. The resultant in any actual case is determined by the relative amplitudes of the two currents. If the resistance is larger than the reactance, the result will be closer to in-phase. A large current flow in the

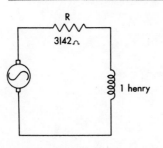

FIG. 1-24.   Schematic of a series resistor (R)–inductor circuit.

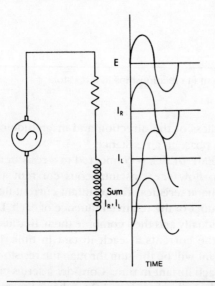

FIG. 1-25.   Current flow in a series resistor-inductor circuit. E = voltage; I_R = current in the resistor; I_L = current in the inductor.

resistor with a small current flow in the coil will give a result much like that of the current in the resistor alone (i.e., close to being in phase with the source). If the inductive reactance is greater than the resistance, the result will be closer to 90° phase lag relative to the source.

To determine the opposition to current flow offered by the coil, one must consider both the construction of the coil and the signal passing through it. If the wires are close together, the lines of force are going to cut more conductors than if the turns are far apart. Also, if there are many turns, the back EMF will be greater because there are many more conductors in which current is induced. Twice as many turns should cause twice the induced current, and so on.

What else might influence the opposition to current flow? The rate at which the EMF is changing direction should also affect the induced current because the lines of force are expanding and collapsing slowly with a *low frequency,* which means that the current will have a chance to build up to some high value before the lines change direction and cause the back EMF to interfere again. Therefore, the frequency at which you are trying to push electrons through a coil influences the opposition to flow.

As noted earlier, this opposition to flow in an inductor is called *inductive reactance* (X_L), and the equation expressing inductive reactance is $X_L = 2\pi fL$, where f is the frequency and L is some measure of the inductance of the coil and is determined by the physical characteristics of the coil. The 2π is a constant. L is measured in henrys, and frequency in hertz. From the equation, we know that an increase in the inductance (L) increases the reactance (X_L), and an increase in the frequency (f) will also increase the reactance. Increasing the size of the coil would increase the inductance; having the voltage source reverse electrical field faster would increase the frequency. Any of the above will increase the opposition to current flow.

The mechanical analog may make this clearer. It is easier to move a small mass than a large mass at a higher rate since a small mass has less opposition to movement. One can move a box of feathers back and forth faster than one can move a refrigerator. Increasing the mass increases the difficulty in increasing the rate of movement. The mass is analogous to the inductance, and the rate of movement is analogous to the frequency. Increasing either increases the opposition to any change.

To return to the circuit in Figure 1-24, let us assume that the voltage source has a frequency of 500 Hz. The EMF is pushing electrons through the resistor; the current would be in phase with the voltage if the inductance were not in the circuit. Likewise, the current would be 90° out of phase with the voltage in the inductor if the inductor were alone in the circuit. Since all the electrons must flow through both the inductor and the resistor, the current flow will have to have the same phase at each point in the circuit.

To determine the magnitude of current flow, the EMF and the resistance values can be plugged into Ohm's law and the current through the resistor can be determined. The same may then be done with the inductive reactance. Following this, the current at each point in time in the resistor is added to the current through the inductor at the same time. Figure 1-24 shows this graphically. The resulting current has a phase angle with the EMF of 45° because the resistance and the inductive reac-

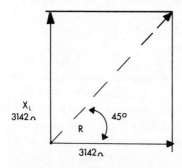

FIG. 1-26.   Phase angle determined with a vector diagram from equal inductive reactance (X_L) and resistance (R) as in Figure 1-24. $X_L = 2\pi(500)(1) = 3,142$ Ω.

tance are equal. If the resistor were larger, the current would be more nearly in phase with the voltage; if smaller, the current would be more nearly 90° out of phase. The vector diagram in Figure 1-26 will provide the same information as the graphing of the waveforms (as in Fig. 1-25) and is much simpler to compute.

To illustrate how the phase angle will vary with varying values of resistance, we will compute the impedance (total opposition to current flow) in three circuits, each of which contains only a resistance and an inductance, choosing three different values for the resistance and keeping the inductance constant. If L = 1 henry, f = 200 Hz, and R equals, in turn, 100 or 1,000 or 10,000, then for R = 100, $X_L = 2\pi fL = (6.28)$ (200)(1) = 1,256.4 Ω. The equation for impedance (Z) is:

$$\begin{aligned} Z = \sqrt{R^2 + X_L^2} &= \sqrt{(100)^2 + 1,579,044} \\ &= \sqrt{10,000 + 1,579,044} \\ &= \sqrt{1,589,044} \\ &= 1,260.7 \ \Omega \end{aligned}$$

That is, with R = 100, notice that the impedance (1,260.7 Ω) is very little different in magnitude from the circuit impedance if the inductance were the only element (1,256.4 Ω) in the circuit.

If the value of R is taken as 1,000, the resulting impedance is equal to 1,605.9.

$$\begin{aligned} Z = \sqrt{R^2 + X_L^2} \\ = \sqrt{1,000^2 + 1,579,044} \\ = 2,579,044 \\ = 1,605.9 \ \Omega \end{aligned}$$

Notice that the current is almost 45° out of phase. It would be exactly 45° if the R (1,000 Ω) were equal to the X_L (1,256.6 Ω), as we would see in Figure 1-24.

In the final case, R = 10,000 and the impedance value is 10,079.0.

$$Z = \sqrt{R^2 + X_L^2}$$
$$= \sqrt{10,000^2 + 1,579,044}$$
$$= \sqrt{101,579,044}$$
$$= 10,079.0 \ \Omega$$

This time the Z is almost exactly the same as R alone, and the phase will be close to that of a resistive circuit, so that current and voltage will be almost in phase.

These three examples allow us to conclude that the phase angle will be a function of the larger value contributing to the impedance. If the R is much larger, the phase will be almost 0, and if the X_L is much larger, the phase will be more nearly 90°.

CAPACITANCE

A capacitor is shown in the schematic in Figure 1-27. The horizontal lines A and B represent metal plates separated by a nonconductor, either air or a nonconducting material, known as the *dielectric.* In reality, capacitors consist of two large sheets of conducting material arranged as a sandwich with an insulator between; the sheets are then rolled into tubes, which allows quite large sheets to be contained in a small area. If wires are connected to each of the sheets and the circuit in Figure 1-27 is connected, consider what happens. Initially, there is an open circuit and no current can flow. In this condition the uncharged plates each have an equal number of electrons. When the switch is closed, there is a momentary surge of current as the excess electrons on the negative side of the battery leave and distribute themselves on the metal plate A to maintain circuit equilibrium. The electrons on both plates space themselves so that they are evenly distributed. (Because electrons are all negatively charged and mutually repellent, they will spread as far from one another as they can, resulting in an even distribution on each plate. All the electrons that the plate connected to the negative side of the battery can hold will have come from the battery, a source of yet higher negative charge.) As the electrons pile up on plate A, the discrepancy in EMF between the plate and battery diminishes until flow stops. The result is an initial surge of current in both connecting wires; that is, electrons flow from the negative pole of the battery to plate A, and electrons are "drained" from plate B and flow to the positive pole of the battery. The two metal plates are now charged—one with an excess of electrons and

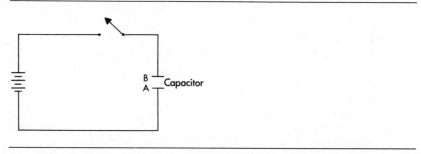

FIG. 1-27.   Schematic of DC circuit with switch, battery, and capacitor.

the other with a lack of electrons, or a positive charge. If the plates were removed from the circuit and connected to a light bulb, the bulb would intially glow as the excess electrons from the negatively charged plate flowed through the bulb to the other plate so as to reach an equilibrium. Then electron flow would stop and the bulb would go out.

A capacitor is analogous to a spring. As pressure is first applied to a compression spring it is easy to move toward further compression, but gets more and more difficult as the spring is further compressed. Compressing the spring stores energy in it, and, if the energy is released, the spring can do some work. In an AC circuit connected to a capacitor, there is no opposition to current flow when the voltage is first applied. As more and more electrons build up on one plate, the opposition increases until the flow stops altogether or the applied voltage changes direction. In the latter case, the current can once again flow easily because the plate that previously lacked electrons now receives them. If the AC is such a low frequency that the push in one direction lasts long enough for sufficient electrons to accumulate on one plate to prevent further flow, the total current flow will be small. If the direction of push changes rapidly, as in a high frequency, flow will be quite large. The rate of change (*frequency*) in direction of the EMF affects the amount of current that can flow. As frequency increases, opposition to flow decreases.

If the plates are quite large, more electrons will be able to accumulate before flow ceases. The larger the plates, the more electrons will be able to accumulate and so the smaller the opposition to current flow. The measure of the amount of storage in a capacitor is called the *capacitance,* which is expressed in farads (F). The number of farads is determined by the construction of the capacitor (e.g., size and spacing of the plates and the dielectric). As capacitance increases, the opposition to flow decreases.

The opposition to electron flow offered by a capacitor is another type of reactance. It is called *capacitive reactance* (X_c) and is expressed by

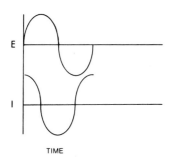

E

I

TIME

FIG. 1-28.   Waveforms of current (I) and voltage (E) in capacitor in AC circuit.

the equation $X_c = 1/(2\pi fc)$, where 2π is the constant, f is the frequency applied, and C is capacitance in farads.

Figure 1-28 is a graph of the voltage (the push) and electron flow in a capacitive circuit. The phase of the current *leads* that of the voltage by 90°. When the EMF reaches a positive state, the current immediately flows at maximum, but, as push continues, the current decreases because of the accumulation of electrons, which tends to repel further flow. When the EMF reverses, current immediately reaches a maximum in the opposite direction and again diminishes.

To examine the effect of the capacitance on the phase angle between current and voltage in a circuit, consider a capacitor of 1 microfarad (μF) in a circuit where f equals 800 Hz and R takes one of three values: 10, 100, or 1,000. The circuit is shown in Figure 1-29. Using the equation for X_c ($X_c = 1/[2\pi fc]$), we find that $X_c = 199.04\ \Omega$. That is, a capacitance of 1 μF offers approximately 200 Ω of capacitive reactance to the flow of a current of 800 Hz. If R $= 10$ and Z $= 199.03\ \Omega$, then:

$$Z = \sqrt{R^2 + X_c^2}$$
$$= \sqrt{(10)^2 + (199.04)^2}$$
$$= \sqrt{100 + 39,616}$$
$$= 199.3\ \Omega$$

This value of Z is almost identical to the impedance in the circuit; therefore, the phase angle of the current derives mostly from the capacitance. If R is changed to 100 Ω we have an impedance of 222.8 Ω.

$$Z = \sqrt{R^2 + X_c^2}$$
$$= \sqrt{(100)^2 + (199.04)^2}$$
$$= \sqrt{49,616}$$
$$= 222.751\ \Omega$$

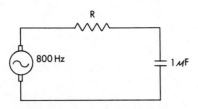

FIG. 1-29.   Series resistor (R)–capacitor circuit.

The R of 1,000 yields a Z of 1,019.6 Ω.

$$Z = \sqrt{R^2 + X_c^2}$$
$$= \sqrt{(1,000)^2 + (199.04)^2}$$
$$= \sqrt{1,039,616}$$
$$= 1,019.6 \ \Omega$$

This value of R (1,000) also yields a phase angle controlled mostly by the greater resistance rather than by the capacitance. To summarize, if we vary R from 10 to 100 to 1,000 and keep X_c constant, we find that Z changes from 199 Ω to 222 Ω to 1,019 Ω. Just as with the inductance, the phase angle will vary depending on the relative values of R with respect to X_c and will approach the angle of the current in the component of largest contribution to the overall opposition to current flow.

THE TOTAL IMPEDANCE EQUATION

Let us consider for a moment the form of the formula for reactance. Reactance is the opposition to the flow of current of varying magnitude. Circuit elements that are reactive are of two types: coils (inductors), the first type, increase their reactance progressively for progressively faster rates of change in current magnitude. That is, their reactance is greater for higher frequencies. Capacitors, the second type, decrease their reactance progressively for progressively faster rates of change in current magnitude; that is, their reactance diminishes progressively for higher frequencies.

To combine all three elements—resistance, inductive reactance, and capacitive reactance—the impedance equation becomes $Z = \sqrt{R^2 + (X_L - X_c)^2}$. Note that in our equation we have the term $(X_L - X_c)^2$ (which you may remember as the equation developed by Pythagorus for calculating the length of the hypotenuse of a right triangle). This really means $[X_L + (-X_c)]^2$, and the $(-X_c)$ appears because the phase of the X_c is 180° from the phase of the X_L. The result would be some cancellation of one by the other, with the cancellation being complete if

$X_L = X_C$. Complete cancellation is a condition known as *resonance,* which is discussed in a later section.

A useful mnemonic for the voltage and current phase relationships in reactances is ELI THE ICEMAN. The first word, ELI, reminds us that E is ahead of I in L (inductance). ICE reminds us that the current (I) leads the voltage (E) in a capacitance.

The same relations can be expressed graphically. Consider first a resistance plus an inductive reactance. The value of the resistance is represented by a line with a length proportional to its value in ohms. The opposition to flow offered by the inductance is represented by a line X_L units (ohms) long, but at 90° to the resistance (because in inductive reactance current lags voltage by 90°, whereas in resistance current and voltage are in phase, so current in an inductor lags current in a resistor by 90°).

To include capacitive reactance, another vector is added 90° out of phase with resistance, but in the opposite direction from X_L (because in capacitive reactance, current leads voltage by 90° and so leads current in a resistor by 90°), or 180° from X_L. Current in capacitive reactance leads by 90° and in an inductive reactance lags by 90° so the current relationship in a circuit having both inductance and capacitance is capacitive current leads inductive current by 180° (Fig. 1-30). The two types of reactance, having opposite voltage-to-current phase relationships, are graphed in opposition to another. In mechanical terms, this states that the opposition to movement of a body is a function of the mass (analogous to inductance), the elasticity (related but not precisely analogous to capacitance), and the friction (analogous to resistance). In mechanics we often use the reciprocal of elasticity, compliance, in the impedance equation. Compliance is analogous to capacitance. Remember that although friction is the only element using up energy, all the elements determine the total opposition; reactances will store and release—but not consume—the energy according to their characteristics.

The concept of reactances storing but not consuming energy has been only implicit up to this point; some expansion may be helpful. When an inductor has a current surge through it, some of the energy is used in creating the electromagnetic force field that builds up around it. So long as the current flows in one direction, the field is maintained and some energy is thereby held in storage. When the field collapses, the energy returns to the circuit. When a capacitor has current flowing into it in one direction, electrons "pile up" on one plate, and this pileup represents a temporary storing of energy in the charging of the capacitor. When the capacitor is discharged, the energy is returned to the circuit.

By way of contrast, when electrons flow through a resistor, some of the energy is being dissipated as heat, so that this energy is no longer available to the circuit. One reason fluorescent bulbs have lower wattage ratings than incandescent bulbs is that fluorescent bulbs "burn cool" and

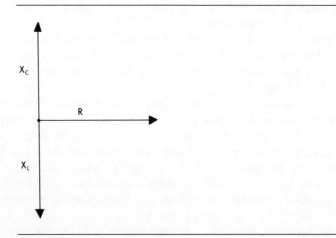

FIG. 1-30. Vectors illustrating relationships of impedance components. R = resistance; X_c = capacitive reactance; X_L = inductive reactance.

do not use up energy as heat in the same way as incandescent bulbs. Therefore a 20-W fluorescent bulb is likely to be brighter than a 100-W incandescent, because the latter is using more energy as heat than it is transducing to light.

A perfect inductor or a perfect capacitor would dissipate no energy, though each would temporarily store some while the circuit was in operation, capturing it as current began to flow and releasing it when the applied current flow ceased. In AC operation, energy is stored in the magnetic field of an inductor or in one plate of a capacitor each half cycle, and returned to the circuit as the current direction changes. It is stored again, in a reversed magnetic field of the inductor or on the opposite plate of the capacitor, as direction of current reverses, and so on for each half cycle.

Using the values we have chosen previously, we can compute the impedance of a circuit as in Figure 1-31. In the circuit, R will take on four successive values: 10, 100, 1,000, and 10,000. Using the vector diagrams or the calculations discussed previously, we would arrive at a series of impedance values of 4,825, 4,826, 4,928, and 11,103.

RESONANCE AND DAMPING

Finally, we will try one more set of values to demonstrate one important characteristic of circuits. Consider the same inductor and capacitor values, but with resistors of 10 and 10,000 Ω and a frequency of 159 Hz. Entering these values into the equations (R = 10 Ω), we find X_L = 999.5 and X_c = 1,001.001. The impedance value then becomes 10.11, and if

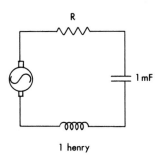

FIG. 1-31.   Series resistor (R)–inductor–capacitor circuit.

we were to connect this in a real circuit, the current would immediately reach an appreciable value. When the single frequency is such that the two reactances are equal, the only opposition to flow is the resistor; so if the resistor value is quite small, the current will reach a very large value. On the other hand, if the resistance is 10,000 Ω, the impedance value would be minimized only to 10,000 when the capacitance and inductance cancel one another out, and current would still be a small value, because of this high impedance.

Figure 1-32 shows what happens to the current value as the frequency is varied. Notice that with the 10-Ω resistor, when the two reactances are equal there is a sharp dip in the impedance curve, which would be reflected as a sharp peak in the current curve. When the resistor is large, the dip is broader and shallower. The point at which the reactances are equal is called the *resonant point.* We define it because at the resonant point in a mechanical system, friction alone can limit the movement of the system. If the friction is great, the turning curve is broad and shallow. If the friction is small, as with a piano string when the damper is not operated, the vibration is large and at one frequency. The energy imparted to the system is exhausted by the friction, so if friction (or R in an electrical circuit) is small, the energy lasts a long time and the piano string hums for quite a while. If the friction is large, as when the damper pedal is pressed, the energy is used up quickly and the string soon stops vibrating.

If a system is set up with an inductance and a capacitance, it is a *tuned system.* There will be some frequency at which the reactances will be equal and the system will have minimal impedance. If the reactance offered by a mass of air is equal to the reactance due to its elasticity, the air will vibrate quite readily.

The impedance of a system will determine the rate of energy flow, with resistance offering a constant opposition to flow and the reactances of-

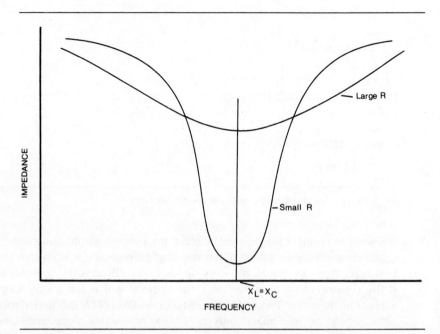

FIG. 1-32.   Change in value of impedance as frequency is varied in resistor-inductor-capacitor circuit for two values of resistance (R).

fering varying amounts of opposition with varying frequency. However, at the point at which the resistances cancel one another, the opposition will be solely resistive. As we have stated, if the resistance in the system is quite small, at the resonance point (that point at which the reactances are equal and, because of their 180° phase difference, cancel each other out) the total opposition is quite small so that the rate of energy flow shows a marked increase. If, on the other hand, the resistance is large, when the reactances cancel, the opposition is still large, so the energy flow does not show much of an increase

Figure 1-32 graphs the relation between impedance and the frequency of an applied signal; the marked dissimilarity of the two curves is due only to the contribution of resistance to the impedance. If R is small, a curve with a sharp peak results. If R is large, the response is broad and not very peaked. The sharpness of the peak is sometimes expressed as the Q of the system; the larger the value of Q, the steeper the response curve. The Q then is a function of the resistance: the smaller the R, the larger the Q. The circuit with a large Q has sharp tuning, and the response changes very sharply. The range of frequencies to which a system will respond is called the *passband;* thus we may say that the edges of the passband are very steep.

The Q of a system is used to advantage in many designs, especially in present-day home music system loudspeakers. Remember that the speakers will exhibit an impedance at various frequencies due to the construction of the elements. Thus, there will be a resonance point at which the response will peak. If the speaker system were a high-Q system, for example, with small resistance of friction, the response would show a sharp peak and the speaker would probably be unpleasant as a music reproducer. To remedy the problems created by the resonance of speakers, designers have provided a large element of acoustic resistance in the system. The result is a lower Q and broader, less peaked, frequency response.

To summarize, the tuning of a system is a function of the impedance, and the peak in the tuning will occur at the point at which the reactances are equal—the resonance point. The steepness of the tuning curve is determined by the relative amount of R to the impedance.

The sensitivity of the device or system will be extremely good within the passband and progressively worse outside it, which may be appropriate for its intended use.

If a flat frequency response is desired, then the circuit should contain few or no reactive elements. If it is impossible to construct the desired circuit with only resistive elements, another way of achieving a flat frequency response is to have a much greater total resistance in the circuit than reactance. The price paid to achieve flat frequency response is the loss in sensitivity, because the high resistance offers great opposition to the flow of signal energy.

Many current-day audio loudspeaker systems have to use highly reactive elements (e.g., loudspeaker coils and magnets with their inductance, loudspeaker cones with their stiffness), but a flat frequency response is desirable. Most often, the construction of a loudspeaker involves a compromise; the loudspeaker enclosure embodies very high resistance so that the system exhibits a better (closer to flat frequency response) characteristic. However, this requires large power amplifiers because much of the power is used to move the signal energy through the high resistance and is dissipated as heat.

We said earlier that there exists an isomorphism (a one-to-one relationship) among acoustics, mechanics, hydraulics, electronics, and mathematics, so that one can consider impedance as applying to auditory testing and measurement. In the middle ear, if an acoustic signal is vibrating the eardrum and ossicles, there will be opposition to movement due to the acoustical elements of mass (inductance), compliance (capacitance), and friction (resistance). The amount of movement and the *instantaneous displacement* (current) compared to the *instantaneous pressure* (voltage) give an indication of the impedance and the values of the reactances and the friction. Practically speaking, in assessing middle ear impedance, the problem is solved backwards; an impedance is measured along with one of the other sides of the right triangle that would yield that impedance, so that all the elemental values can be determined.

The fundamental elements controlling energy flow in the electrical domain are the reactances (inductance and capacitance) and resistance. The reactances differ from the resistance elements because their opposition to current flow is a function of the frequency, whereas resistance elements offer an opposition to energy flow that is independent of frequency.

In each of the other energy domains, there are elements analogous to inductance, capacitance, and resistance. In the mechanical domain, for example, the analogs are inertia (which is analogous to inductance and comes about because of the massiveness of a body), compliance (which is analogous to capacitance and is the result of the lack of springiness of a body), and friction, respectively. However, most times it is difficult in the mechanical domain to construct an element having a particular amount of compliance without that element also embodying some mass and, perhaps, some friction also, whereas it is relatively easy to construct electrical elements embodying the desired amount of one elemental quantity with virtually no influence on either of the other two elements.

Comparable statements can be made about the domains of acoustics and hydraulics. In these the elemental quantities (those analogous to the reactances and resistances) cannot as easily be configured independently of one another in a device as their analogs can be configured in the electrical domain. Therefore, one can easily build an analog in the electrical domain for any device or structure in any of the other domains, but we cannot as easily go the other way. The confounding of elemental quantities (reactances and resistances) in the domains other than the electrical makes the electrical the medium of choice for modeling all the domains.

An important reason for transducing most phenomena into the electrical domain is that the human being is not able to make judgments about sound phenomena that occur over too short or too long a timespan. It is desirable, in some few instances, to speed up phenomena so that changes over time (e.g., changes in vocal quality with age) can be assessed more sensitively. However, most often we desire to slow down phenomena to bring them into the appropriate range for assessment. The electrical domain, with its ability to store signals and to reproduce them with a different time scale (as in computer processing) becomes the medium of choice for these reasons.

As a result of this, we most often transduce from the primary domain in which a phenomenon occurs into the electrical domain for the purposes of manipulating the energy of the signal and for measuring it. Often, because we become familiar with and comfortable about phenomena in the electrical domain, we tend to work in this domain even when

neither the experimental purpose nor aspects of human sensitivity requires it.

Moreover, it is important to note that while experimenters sometimes
assume the electronic domain to be error-free, there are inherent problems (discussed in later chapters) even in electronic media, and the experimenter should pay close attention to the basic physical principles
involved in any domain. For example, there are limits to the frequency
response, the range of sound intensities, and even the duration of sounds
when using magnetic recording. The physical limitations of a system,
however, can also be used to the benefit of a specific hardware application.

As we shall discuss, any meter that moves a pointer arm mechanically
across a calibrated meter dial will exhibit inertia, so that it is slow to
move and slow to stop; that is, it will lag behind sudden increases or
decreases in signal energy. This means that changes occurring faster than
some nominal value will be too fast for the meter and will therefore be
outside its frequency response range. As we shall also discuss, however,
sometimes we prefer that a meter not be able to show rapid changes but
instead show minor changes in quantity and give only some slowly
changing average values. In these cases, we make use of the inertia of the
meter to derive just the average value desired, with the meter being too
slow to follow the more rapid variations. The point remains that whether
we capitalize on the mechanical inadequacies or not, the inadequacies
are inherent to any device in the mechanical domain because of the nature of inertial forces in bodies of any mass.

Impedance-Matching

The efficiency of coupling—of transferring energy with or without a
change in medium—is related to the degree of matching of the characteristics of the input to a transducer and the transducer's output (or the
matching of the characteristics of the output from any device and the
input to any other device to which it is coupled). The matching or mis-
matching of coupled elements is called *impedance-matching,* and because it is so central to all considerations of energy transfer, it is to the
subject of impedance-matching that we now turn.

To make this concept somewhat clearer, consider an electronic circuit
in which we are attempting to provide power to a source. Power is equal
to the voltage times the current. We will neglect any phase difference
between the voltage and the current, as occurs in reactive circuits, and
consider only resistances. Assume that an amplifier is driving a loudspeaker. The amplifier has been designed so that 50 V appears across the
output and the output active elements provide 1 A of current. The

power, then, is 50 W. The designer has provided that the 50 V will appear across 50 Ω, hence the 1 A (Ohm's law again: E = I × R, or 50 V = 50 Ω × 1 A). This means that if 50 Ω is connected across the output there will be 50 W of power. Assume, however, that 100 Ω is connected across the output. Ohm's law then would show that we have only 25 W because the current would be 50 V = 100 Ω × 0.5 A. The power is equal to 50 V × 0.5 A, which equals 25 W. We have not coupled the maximum amount of available signal to the load. In order to have the maximum amount of signal coupled, the impedances must be equal. If they are not, then either the current or the voltage will be less, which means that the power will be less. For this reason, it is important to remember to match impedances when coupling power from one place to another.

At this point it might be well to mention that it is not necessary to match impedance when coupling voltage from one place to another. If a circuit provides a given voltage output, and a load (i.e., a second circuit of another device) is connected across that circuit, the load will be in parallel and, as you will recall, voltages are equal in all elements of a parallel circuit. A mismatch will cause no problem if a load that is added is not so sufficiently small that it changes the operating characteristic of the source. However, if an amplifier has been designed to provide a specific voltage across the output impedance of the device and a much smaller resistance is placed across that impedance, the total impedance seen by the source will be much less than the value for which the circuit is designed, which can be a problem.

To make this clear, consider Figure 1-33. Here an amplifier with an internal output impedance of 100 Ω is connected to a 100-Ω load. The two impedances are in parallel and the total impedance is 50 Ω: $R_t = R_1R_2/(R_1 + R_2) = 100 \times 100/(100 + 100) = 50$. This means that the circuit is not operating into 100 Ω anymore and the design parameters have been violated. To avoid this, if 1,000 Ω is connected as the load, the total impedance will be 100 × 1,000/(100 + 1,000) = 90.9. Better yet, connect 10,000 Ω as the load. The total impedance is 100 × 10,000/ 10,100, or 99.0 Ω. Thus the connection of the load has not changed the operating parameters of the circuit. We have discussed this in some detail because it has been our experience that students often assume that the impedances must always be matched. In this case, when voltage only is being coupled, impedance-matching would not be desirable.

In cases where impedance-matching is a requirement, and the source and the load cannot be changed, then transformers or L and T pads are used. These two devices will also be discussed in specific chapters.

An important caveat that appears to be contrary to the previous discussion of impedance-matching must be inserted at this point. Because of the design and construction of most modern semiconductor power amplifiers, the output impedance of the unit appears not to be fixed and the maximum power output of such an amplifier increases as the imped-

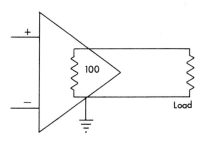

FIG. 1-33.   Schematic of amplifier with 100 Ω of output impedance connected to 100-Ω load.

ance of the connected speakers decreases. In general, most units will deliver their maximum power when connected to very low impedance speakers (e.g., 4 Ω) and quite a bit less with 16 Ω speakers. In these cases, it is best to consult the manufacturer's specifications and connect the proper value of impedance at the output. The engineering reasons for all this are somewhat beyond the scope of the present book.

Suggested Reading

Benade, A. H.   *Horns, Strings, and Harmony.* Garden City, NY: Doubleday, 1960.

Beranek, L. L.   *Acoustic Measurements.* New York: Wiley, 1962.

Borden, G. J., and Harris, K. S.   *Speech Science Primer.* Baltimore: Williams & Wilkins, 1984.

Crowhurst, N. H.   *Basic Audio.* New York: Rider, 1959.

Durant, J. D., and Lovrinic, J. H.   *Bases of Hearing Science.* Baltimore: Williams & Wilkins, 1984.

Malmstadt, H. V., and Enke, C. G.   *Electronics for Scientists.* New York: Benjamin, 1963.

Minifie, F. D., Hixon, T. J., and Williams, F.   *Normal Aspects of Speech, Hearing and Language.* Englewood Cliffs, N.J.: Prentice-Hall, 1978.

Roederer, J. G.   *Introduction to the Physics and Psychophysics of Music.* New York: Springer-Verlag, 1974.

Ryder, J. D.   *Engineering Electronics.* New York: McGraw-Hill, 1957.

VanValkenburgh, Nooger, and Neville, Inc.   *Basic Electronics.* New York: Rider, 1955.

II. Manipulation of
the Electrical Signal

2. Filters: Frequency Control

General Principles

In the previous chapter it was made abundantly clear that reactive elements exhibit different impedances at different frequencies (see also Chap.5). Advantage is taken of this characteristic in a series of devices called *filters*. The speech system provides an excellent example of filtering. Filtering is responsible for the differentiation of speech sounds. That is, the source of power for the voiced sounds is a vibrating column of air, which is set into motion by two flaps of vibrating tissue, the vocal cords. All voiced sounds begin with this same vibrating column of air. How, then, are we able to produce sounds that have different acoustical characteristics? By filtering. The vibration from the vocal folds contains many different frequencies. The vocal cavities, depending on their size and shape, support the vibration of the air at some frequencies and attenuate the vibration at other frequencies. The result, in the case of vowel sounds, is a series of bands of energy within certain frequency regions, the formants. Each vowel has a different pattern of formants. How do we know that each vowel contains a pattern of formants? We take a speech sound and feed it into a set of filters. The filters can be tuned to allow passage of only specific frequencies. If we adjust the filter to a specific frequency, measure the output, and find a great deal of energy there, we can be relatively certain that the specific frequency is present. By this means we can analyze any sound into its frequency components (i.e., successively adjust a filter to different frequencies and read the output on a meter).

There are several kinds of filters, both active and passive with several quite different functions, found in equipment. Central to describing filters is the transfer function.

THE TRANSFER FUNCTION

The *transfer function,* often used to describe the operation of an electronic device, is a graph of the output of the device with respect to amplitude and frequency, assuming an input of all frequencies at equal amplitude. A linear amplifier would simply produce an output whose spectrum was unchanged from the input except for an increase in amplitude equal to the gain of the amplifier. A filter, as we shall see in the next section, will not produce a constant output regardless of frequency, but will exhibit a great deal more amplitude at some frequencies (the passband) than at others. The *passband* is the range of frequencies that a system will pass. The passband of a device is the range of frequencies from the lower point at which the output is one-half the maximum power (3 dB less) to the upper frequency at which the power has dropped to one-half. Figure 2-1 should make this clear.

OPERATING PRINCIPLES

Before discussing specific filter designs, we will review our discussion of reactance and the combining of resistance (R), capacitance (C), and inductance (L). If two resistors are connected in series and a voltage is placed across them, part of the voltage will be dropped across one resistor and the remainder across the other. This will happen regardless of frequency. If one of the resistors is replaced with a capacitor, part of the voltage will be dropped across the resistor and part across the capacitive reactance. Recall from the discussion of impedance that as the frequency increases, the reactance of the capacitor decreases. This is equivalent to having two resistors in series with one of the resistors changing value as the frequency changes. If the frequency increases, the situation would be similar to replacing one of the resistors in our original circuit with resistors of successively smaller value. As the value of the resistor decreases, the voltage drop across it decreases. If we graph the voltage drop across the capacitor as the frequency changes, we might obtain a graph of the transfer function similar to Figure 2-2. If we place a device across the capacitor that converts the voltage across the capacitor into a sound, the loudness of the sound decreases as we increase frequency. If, however, we place the sound producer across the resistor, the sound increases in loudness because more and more of the voltage is dropped across the resistor as we increase frequency. (If it is not dropped across the capacitor, it must be dropped across the resistor. To reiterate: the total voltage must be dropped across the two elements.) The amount dropped across each element is a function of the proportion of the impedance contributed by that element. If the capacitor is exhibiting less reactance, then it must be contributing a smaller proportion of the total impedance.

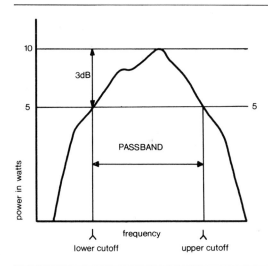

FIG. 2-1.   Transfer function of a bandpass filter.

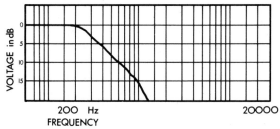

A

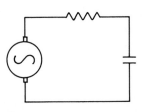

B

FIG. 2-2.   A. Magnitude (in volts) of response of circuit shown in (B) changes with varying frequency. B. Capacitance circuit.

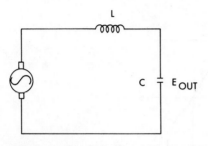

FIG. 2-3.   A series AC circuit with a capacitor (C) and an inductor (L). E_{OUT} = output voltage.

Types of Filters

PASSIVE FILTERS

If you refer to Figure 2-2, you will note that the reactance decreases by half for each doubling of the frequency. This means a halving of the voltage that is dropped across the capacitor for each doubling of the frequency. Recall that half the voltage is equal to a change of 6 dB, and that a doubling or halving of frequency is a change of 1 octave, and we can predict that if we graph the voltage output versus frequency we will find that it changes by 6 dB per octave. When the output is taken across the capacitor we said that the signal decreases as the frequency increases. The result is less high-frequency response. This is the phenomenon associated with a bass tone control on an amplifier. Conversely, if the output is across the resistor, the signal increases with frequency, which is equivalent to a treble tone control.

Consider placing a capacitor and inductor in series and determining the voltage across each as the frequency is increased, as shown in Figure 2-3. From Chapter 1 we know that as frequency increases the reactance of the inductor will increase, so that the circuit could be simulated by replacing the inductor with successively larger resistors as frequency increases and the capacitor with successively smaller resistors. The result would be a change of voltage of 6 dB per octave for the inductor and 6 dB per octave for the capacitor. Thus, output would change by 12 dB per octave for the circuit. In the case of a filter the steepness with which the frequencies roll off outside the passband is considered an important parameter. The edges of the graph of the transfer function are called the *skirts,* and the slope of these skirts may be an important consideration in the design of a filter. The *slope* is the rate of change of amplitude with frequency. Usually the figure is in terms of decibels per octave.

Thus far we have discussed only *passive filters.* In general, passive filters are not capable of rolloffs of much greater than 18 dB per octave.

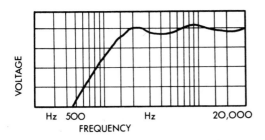

FIG. 2-4.   The output voltage from a highpass filter for a constant input voltage and varying frequency.

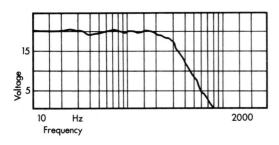

FIG. 2-5.   The output voltage from a lowpass filter for a constant input voltage and varying frequency.

Passive filters are devices that contain frequency-sensitive elements but no active elements (e.g., no vacuum tubes or semiconductors). Therefore, the use of the filter will automatically attenuate the signal level as the filter will offer some impedance to the signal. Further, the filter may be highpass, lowpass, bandpass, or band-reject. Figure 2-4 shows the response of a *highpass* filter, and Figure 2-5 shows a *lowpass* response. A highpass filter offers minimal impedance to the transfer of frequencies above some value (called the *low-frequency cutoff),* but increasingly greater impedance to frequencies below the cutoff. A lowpass filter is the complement of a highpass filter in offering minimal impedance below the cutoff and increasingly greater impedance above it. If these two filters are connected together in series the result will be a bandpass filter, which is a device that allows a specific band of frequencies to pass through between the low-frequency cutoff and the high-frequency cutoff. This band of frequencies is called the *passband.* Figure 2-6 shows a typical filter and the controls. The filter shown can be operated as a highpass, lowpass, or bandpass filter, depending on the control settings, which will be described later. The band-reject (or *notch*) filter is one that passes *all*

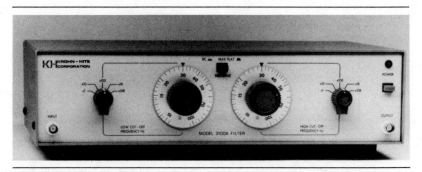

FIG. 2-6.   A filter that can be operated as a highpass, lowpass, or a bandpass filter.

frequencies, *except* a band. This type of filter has many uses, the most common being to eliminate some noise that is obscuring the signal of interest but that is not part of that signal.

When the multiplier dial is used, the value on the frequency dial is multiplied by the value on the multiplier dial to obtain the cutoff frequency. The cutoff frequency of a filter is a frequency arbitrarily selected as the nominal value. It could be the highest (for a lowpass) or lowest (for a highpass) value passed with minimal attenuation—before entering the zone of frequencies being rejected. Conventionally, it is that value on the slope of the filter (i.e., in the region where its response is diminishing) where only half of the power is passed. The half-power point is also called the 3 dB down point (see Fig. 2-1).

Consider an amplifier passing all frequencies equally, that is, having a flat frequency response. If this amplifier feeds a white noise to a highpass filter with a cutoff of 300 Hz, for example, the input of the filter will be an equal amplitude (or equal power) spectrum (as in Fig. 2-7), but the output will resemble Figure 2-8. The filter is labeled as having a 300 Hz– cutoff because the output is down 3 dB at 300 Hz from peak output at other frequencies.

The Time Constant

The time constant (TC) of a series-reactive circuit is a useful parameter in specifying performance. If the circuit in Figure 2-9 is connected, the capacitor will begin to charge. The rate at which it will charge is a function of the value of both the resistor and the capacitor. Initially, the capacitor offers no opposition to electron flow, and the flow is determined solely by the value of the resistor. However, as the capacitor charges it becomes more and more difficult to accumulate electrons because of those already present. The TC of a series resistor-capacitor (RC) circuit is defined as the length of time required for the capacitor to charge to

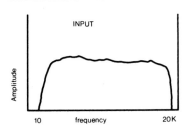

FIG. 2-7.   **Typical white noise spectrum showing essentially equal amplitude at
all frequencies in the audio range.**

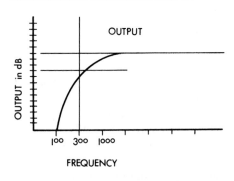

FIG. 2-8.   **The output voltage of a highpass filter with a cutoff at 300 Hz.**

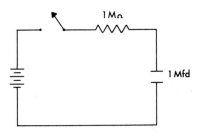

FIG. 2-9.   **A resistor-capacitor circuit with a 1-second time constant.**

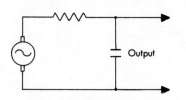

FIG. 2-10.   A resistor-capacitor lowpass filter.

63.7% of the total applied voltage and is equal to R × C. In Figure 2-9, this would be 1 second. How is this determined? When the circuit is first connected, the current flow is equal to E/R because the capacitor offers no opposition. If the capacitor never offered any opposition, it would charge to the full voltage in one time constant. But the capacitor begins to offer opposition as a voltage drop develops across it and, thus, less across the resistance. This means current decreases. The current decreases at an exponential rate so that, at the end of one time constant, the charge is 63.7% of the total. Again, TC = C × (E/I) (TC = R × C, R = E/I, so TC = C × E/I). That is, the TC of a circuit in seconds equals the resistance in ohms times the capacitance in farads. (The TC for a series RL circuit—the time necessary for it to charge to 63.7% of its maximum—equals R/L.)

This computation can be useful in determining, for example, the maximum frequency that can be applied to a combination of R and C. If the TC is so great that the capacitor never charges to the full value before the signal changes phase, then less than the full AC signal will appear across the capacitor. The result is filtering. If the circuit in Figure 2-10 is connected, the voltage across C will be very close to full value for slowly varying signals, but low for signals that last only a short time. This is a lowpass filter. Connected as in Figure 2-11, the capacitor never charges to the full value for high frequencies because current does not flow in one direction for as long as the time constant. That means that most of the voltage appears across R at high frequencies. At low frequencies, conversely, the capacitor can charge, so the voltage drop is greater there and, hence, lesser across R. The result is a highpass filter.

ACTIVE FILTERS

An *active filter* consists of amplifiers tuned to various frequencies so that the amplifier passes only specific frequencies. The result is usually a cheaper way than passive filters in complicated and expensive multielement designs to obtain a steeper slope to the filter characteristics.

The active filter also allows greater variation in input and output impedances while retaining its design characteristics. The passive filter,

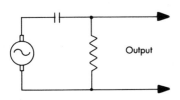

FIG. 2-11.   A resistor-capacitor highpass filter.

on the other hand, varies in impedance with frequency; consequently, the loads connected at the output must be within a specified impedance range for the tuning of the filter to be as labeled. The active filter contains amplifiers whose input impedance is high, so that quite a wide range of input impedances may be used. Also, the output impedance is low, and this allows various loads to be connected without adversely affecting the tuning since there are amplifiers before and after the tuning elements (these are called *buffer amplifiers* and are commonly used to prevent external characteristics from adversely affecting circuitry having stringent impedance parameters).

Passive filters, because they operate by attenuating certain frequencies, may introduce some loss of signal even in the passband. This is called the *insertion loss.* An active filter can compensate for insertion loss by providing some gain in the passband.

Uses of Filters

HUM FILTERS

A filter having a characteristic of easily passing energy below 100 Hz (a 100-Hz lowpass filter) is frequently connected from the input of a piece of equipment to ground. Energy of lower frequencies now goes to ground instead of entering the equipment. The purpose served by the filter is to remove any 60-Hz "hum" from the desired signal (the 60-Hz energy is often introduced by electromagnetic input from the stray magnetic fields of wires and the like in the vicinity). In this way, much of what could be a troubling noise is removed from any later analysis at little or no loss of signal energy.

FILTERS IN THE SPECTROGRAPH

The sound spectrograph, like many other pieces of equipment for speech analysis, makes use of a filter that is a variable bandpass, having a constant band width but a variable center frequency. The use of the filter with a repeated sample of speech (from an endless loop of recording tape) allows analysis of the frequency components in a short sample of speech (i.e., the relative energy at each frequency) for purposes of analyzing voice quality or other speech characteristics.

MASKING FILTERS

Masking in audiometry is another situation in which filters are routinely used. The sensitivity of one ear is tested while a narrow band of noise, centered at the test frequency, is delivered to the contralateral ear (the ear not under test). In this way, we may ensure that the ear under test is, in fact, being appraised, since possible cross-hearing is precluded by the masking created by the presentation of a filtered noise to the contralateral ear.

TONE CONTROL

Tone controls consist of electronic components whose opposition to current flow varies as a function of frequency, so that they offer minimal opposition at some frequencies but more as the frequency is varied higher or lower. The bass control offers more opposition to high frequencies than it does to low frequencies; therefore, the output sounds as if the low frequencies had been boosted. The converse is true for the treble control.

WAVE ANALYSIS

There are devices called *wave analyzers* that are typically constructed as a series of filters whose outputs can be displayed either simultaneously or, by rapidly switching from one to another, individually. Wave analyzers allow easy analysis and display of complex waves such as speech waves or evoked-response waveforms.

FREQUENCY EQUALIZATION

For some laboratory purposes, a shaping of the frequency spectrum may be desirable. For example, one might desire to smooth the response of a loudspeaker system for listening tests to be conducted in a highly reverberant room by reducing some of the higher frequency output. Alternatively, one might desire to simulate a hearing loss by manipulating a complex signal to introduce a signal loss matching the threshold shift.

In these cases as well as others, a multiband filter system (equalizer) is used. In the typical equalizer used for laboratory purposes, each filter band will be of some fixed value (frequently found values are one-third octave bands and full-octave bands), and the attenuation in each band can be set independently. Frequently, such pieces of equipment are constructed so that the attenuator control is a variable resistor that is moved vertically to increase or decrease the level in that band (variable resistors will be discussed in somewhat more detail in the following chapter). The face of the device displays the frequency response curve that is imposed because each of the controls appears to be a spot on a frequency response graph.

Still another variety of equalizer is found on home stereo systems. This circuit design yields a shaping of the entire frequency spectrum so as to compensate for the smaller dynamic range of the ear or for the lower and higher frequencies more than for the midfrequencies. Without the loudness equalization, the low and high frequencies would become inaudible as the overall level of the entire spectrum was reduced. This equalizer circuit delivers greater midfrequency than high or low frequency attenuation so as to retain audibility for the entire spectrum.

Clinical Applications

This chapter has examined devices that shape the frequency response of any signal of interest, sometimes to obtain some desired frequency characteristic (e.g., to "shape" a flat frequency response or to eliminate some portion of the frequency band). For other situations, the user may wish to have local control over the frequency response so as to be able to vary it at will (e.g., to increase the low frequency, or bass, or the high frequency, or treble, response of a loudspeaker). All of these uses arise from the frequency-selective properties of reactive elements, with coils or inductances favoring low frequencies and offering significant opposition to higher frequencies, and condensors or capacitors favoring high frequencies and offering significant opposition to lower frequencies.

At this point we might consider two very simple applications of filters to laboratory situations. One of the most common occurs when one is attempting to use some equipment that results in a low-frequency hum at the output. Of course, an attempt should be made to determine what is causing the hum, but if the cause cannot be discovered then a highpass filter might be inserted into the line and its controls set to filter out the noise. This might even be used when trying to use a tape recording that has been made under less than ideal conditions. In this case the tape would be dubbed from one machine to another, passing the signal through a filter between the machines. The hum is often at 60 Hz or 120 Hz, the latter originating in the power supply of some equipment.

Another use of filters is in locating a specific frequency. For example, one might be looking for a particular frequency in an electroencephalographic record. In this case a bandpass filter set to the frequency region of interest might be used.

Finally, filters may be used to improve the quality of a sound system. If a system is being played in a very highly damped room (i.e., a room with almost no reverberation), high frequencies may be attenuated to the point that they are masked by the low frequencies. In this case, a highpass filter might be used to attenuate some of the low frequencies and bring them down to the level of the high frequencies. This, of course, is exactly what the tone control on reproducers accomplishes.

Suggested Reading

Crowhurst, N. H.   *Basic Audio.* New York: Rider, 1959.

Everest, F. A.   *Acoustic Techniques for Home and Studio.* Blue Ridge Summit, PA: TAB Books, 1984.

Lancaster, D.   *Active Filter Cookbook.* Indianapolis: Sams, 1975.

Malmstadt, H. V., and Enke, C. G.   *Electronics for Scientists.* New York: Benjamin, 1963.

Tucker, D. G.   *Elementary Electrical Network Theory.* New York: Macmillan, 1964.

3. Attenuators: Amplitude Control

This chapter deals with the control of the intensity of a signal and methods of varying the intensity in predetermined units. These attenuating devices are, of course, the heart of audiometers, but also appear as volume controls on radios and gain controls on amplifiers. The student may need to review material on Ohm's law (see Chap. 1) and decibel notation as discussed in *Bases of Hearing Science* by Durrant and Lovrinic or in *Normal Aspects of Speech, Hearing, and Language* by Minifie, Hixon, and Williams (see Suggested Reading).

Amplitude is one of the primary dimensions of an audio signal and often must be controlled and varied. In some applications, the variation must be precisely controlled, as in an audiometer or sound level meter; in other applications, some ability to vary loudness for comfort is desirable. And finally, in the majority of cases, the only requirement is for a device that will decrease the amount of signal fed from one (portion of a) circuit to another. This device is often given the misnomer *volume control*, but the preferred label is *gain control*. All of these devices are attenuators.

Amplifiers will be discussed in a later chapter, but for now, consider a device that is capable of increasing the voltage fed into an amplifier. The product of the voltage at the output divided by the input voltage is called the *gain*. For example, 1 V is fed into a device and 10 V appears at the output. In this case the gain is a factor of 10, because we are dealing with a voltage ratio of 10 to 1, or 20 dB. If two of these devices are connected in series so that the output of one is fed to the input of another and each has a gain of 10, the result is a gain of 100 (10 × 10) or, in decibels, 40 dB.

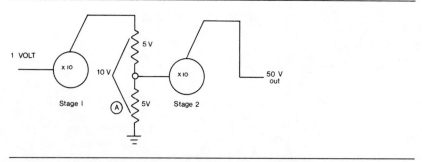

FIG. 3-1.   A voltage divider between stages of an amplifier.

Gain Controls

VOLTAGE DIVIDERS

If a gain of something less than 100 but more than 10 were desired, the gain control would be used. For example, if this series circuit were intended to feed a device requiring only 50 V at its input, a full gain of 100 would provide 100 V (i.e., the 1-V input is increased to 100 V), which would overload the following unit. To decrease the gain of the circuit, two resistors of equal value could be placed in series on the output of stage 1, as shown in Figure 3-1. The input to the second stage would be connected to the junction of the two resistors so that the voltage will be reduced before reaching the second stage, resulting in a gain of only 50 across the two stages. The full 10-V output from the first stage appears across the two resistors. Since the resistors are of equal value, 5 V are dropped across each resistor. The 5 V across the lower resistor (A) are all the second stage "sees." The second stage, like the first, has a gain of 10, so the resultant output is 50 V. The resistor circuit illustrated is a type of *attenuator.* The result is a gain of 50 instead of 100; thus the name "gain control."

STEP ATTENUATORS

If, instead of two resistors, a switch is installed with several pairs of resistors whose values are selected so that differing amounts of voltage could appear at the second stage, the gain of the circuit could be controlled in steps. This is called a *step attenuator* or *ladder network.* For example, consider Figure 3-2. In this case, when the switch is at position 1 the gain is 50. When the switch moves to position 2, 8 V is dropped across resistor B so that only 2 V appears across the input of the second stage. Now the output is only 20 V and the gain of the circuits is 20. Step 3 results in a gain of only 10. Note that the gain is a function of the ratio of the two resistance values. If the resistance values were chosen so that the gain varied logarithmically, the result would be a decibel attenuator.

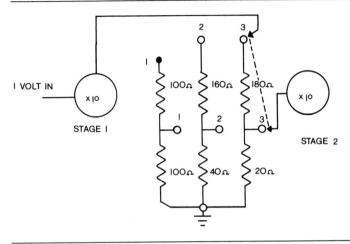

FIG. 3-2.   Schematic of step attenuator gain control.

Switch position	1	2	3
First stage	10	10	10
Input to 2	5	2	1
Output	50	20	10

In some rare cases the gain is varied in this way, as in some meters or in audiometers.

POTENTIOMETERS

In the usual amplifier, the gain is controlled in a continuous fashion by using a *variable resistor,* sometimes called a *potentiometer.* Figure 3-3 shows a variable resistor. Note that there is a resistor element, which is either a strip coated with the same sort of carbon compound used in fixed resistors or a strip of insulating material around which is wrapped resistance wire. This wire consists of alloys yielding various amounts of resistance per foot. There is also a movable wiper that can be positioned at various points along the resistor elements so that, in essence, two resistors are formed, one on either side of the wiper. That is, each end of the resistor is tied into the circuit, but the desired voltage is picked off between one end and the wiper so that the voltage varies as the wiper moves. Because the wiper can be located anywhere along the resistor, it is possible to have an infinite number of pairs of resistors so that the voltage can be divided infinitely. The potentiometer is the gain control found in almost all amplifiers.

Recently there has been one small problem associated with the gain control. It is sometimes difficult to associate a given level with a given rotation of the gain control. To overcome this small operational problem,

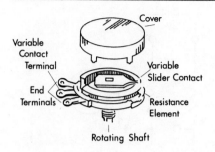

FIG. 3-3.   An exploded view of a wire-wound variable resistor.

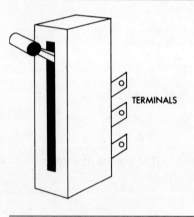

FIG. 3-4.   Slider variable resistor.

variable resistances are made in which the element consists of a strip of resistive material and the wiper slides along it in a straight line. Thus, the control moves only back and forth or up and down. In adjusting the channels of an amplifier, this straight line movement results in much more precise alignment. Figure 3-4 shows one of these new controls.

TAPERS

The *taper* of a gain control is also an important factor. Recall that the ear does not respond in a linear fashion when judging loudness as amplitude is varied. That is, decreasing the amplitude by half does not result in half-loudness. Rather, the auditory system responds more in a logarithmic fashion—hence our use of decibels. When the gain control is turned 10° (i.e., one-ninth of a quarter turn) in a simple variable resistor—one in which the resistance increases linearly with length from one end to the

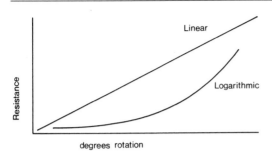

FIG. 3-5.   Tapers for two common gain controls.

wiper—the *amplitude* of the signal will be decreased the same amount, no matter where the 10° occurs in the total, but not the loudness because loudness does not decrease equally with amplitude at different frequencies. As a result, if the loudness of the signal is to vary consistently with consistent rotation of the control, the resistance must vary logarithmically. To provide equal loudness controls, there are variable resistors designed in which resistance varies logarithmically as the control is rotated. There is much more resistance for a 10° rotation at one end of the control than for an equal rotation at the other. Figure 3-5 shows how the voltage-dividing action takes place with the linear control and with the logarithmic control. The variation in resistance with rotation of the control is called the *taper;* the control on the left of the figure has a *linear taper* while the control on the right has an *audio taper.*

LOUDNESS CONTROLS

It might be well to point out at this time that controls that are labeled *loudness* on amplifiers have one further refinement beyond the taper. Recall that the auditory system does not respond equally in loudness at all frequencies for equal amplitude of the signal. The trough-shaped threshold curve of Sivian and White in any audiology text illustrates this. However, at more intense levels the ear begins to respond equally so that, for loud sounds of equal amplitude, the loudness judgment is almost equal. If one were listening to music at a loud level, for example, one would hear all the instruments with approximately equal loudness. If one were to attenuate the signal, however, the frequencies at the extremes of the frequency range would appear to decrease in loudness more than those in the middle. This results in the spectrum of the music changing with the signal level. To avoid this, a gain control has been constructed that is designed to attenuate the middle of the spectrum more than the extremes. At very soft levels the resultant spectrum is almost a mirror-image of the threshold curve. Figure 3-6 shows a hypothetical gain func-

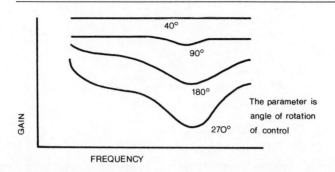

FIG. 3-6.   Variation in gain as a function of frequency for four different positions of a loudness control.

tion for a loudness control. The result is that at low levels the low and high frequencies are somewhat more intense than the middle frequencies. When such a complex gain control is used, the auditory system does not perceive any change in spectrum with attenuation of the signal. Admittedly, use of such a gain control distorts the acoustic signal so that it is not desirable in other than an aesthetic context. What must be kept in mind, then, is that a loudness control is not only a gain control but also a variable filter.

AUDIOMETER ATTENUATORS

The audiometer attenuator is an example of a combination of the two types of attenuators we have discussed thus far: the step attenuator and the variable resistor. The reason for this combination will be obvious when one considers that in order to cover the entire 110- or 120-dB range necessary on the audiometer with a step attenuator there would be 22 or more switch positions, depending upon the size of the steps. While this is possible, the selection of the resistors would be a difficult and time-consuming as well as an expensive task. To avoid this, a special control is used, consisting of a wire-wound resistor with taps along its length. That is, at perhaps ten points along the resistor, connections are made to fixed resistors that are connected as in Figure 3-7. The arrangement appears to be a combination of the voltage divider network, but with one leg connected to a continuously variable resistor; the wiper then selects resistances in between to provide 2- or 5-dB steps. This type of attenuator is much larger than the usual variable gain control because of the precision with which it must be wound and because of the several taps and sets of fixed resistors.

The subject of attenuators is one that seldom concerns the clinician but all too frequently faces the researcher who is connecting a series of

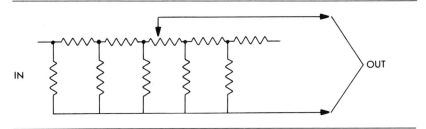

FIG. 3-7.   Schematic of attenuator used in some audiometers.

components together for some laboratory purpose. Because attenuators are important and also because the subject is too frequently given short shrift in elementary or even advanced texts on electronics, we are devoting more attention to it than is usual. The section that follows discusses attenuators only very generally. The Appendix provides the information necessary to design a wide variety of attenuators.

Attenuators are frequently used to supply a constant load resistance to a circuit. For example, some amplifiers are designed so that they operate within published specifications, particularly with reference to harmonic distortion, only if they are terminated in or near some specified impedance. A common way of supplying an optimum impedance is to load or terminate the amplifier with an attenuator constructed of resistances only, and so constructed that the load resistance to the amplifier remains constant even though the amount of attenuation may vary.

At times an attenuator is used between two pieces of equipment so that each piece of equipment is terminated (or loaded) in its own optimal impedance, which may be different from the other piece's optimal impedance. For example, one may desire to hook earphones of 10-Ω impedance to an amplifier that requires a load impedance of 600 Ω. An attenuator is required that will present a 600-Ω load to the amplifier and 10-Ω source to the earphones; additionally, the attenuator may have to introduce sufficient attenuation that the earphones are not burned out because too much power is delivered to them.

For other uses, one may require an attenuator that will match the impedance of each of the pieces of equipment to which it is connected but may desire that minimal attenuation be introduced.

Attenuators may be used in equipment that is unbalanced, with one side of the equipment being at ground potential, or in equipment that is balanced, with both sides being at some potential difference from ground. This means that there are two types of attenuators, *balanced* and *unbalanced.* (The more common condition is that of unbalanced circuitry.)

Attenuators in Circuits

Given the design of various types of attenuators we should now consider how they can best be placed in the various circuits to result in significant changes in operating characteristics. Take, for example, the simple gain control in the amplifier. Because electronic circuits are not perfect, there will be some noise (electrical disturbance not part of the signal) introduced into each stage of an amplifier. Transistors may generate heat, which causes random motion of electrons that is added to the motion of electrons caused by the signal input. Thus the output will contain the electron motion due to the input signal and also the random motion due to heat, among other causes. Furthermore, each stage of an amplifier will have some amount of noise. This means that each stage of an amplifier will amplify the noise generated by each preceding stage. If we were to connect the gain control at the output, then the signal, as well as the noise, would be decreased in value. The result is an attenuation of the noise—a very desirable result. However, if the input signal is so strong that the amplifier is receiving too much signal, each stage may distort the signal. To eliminate this, the gain control could be placed at the input. Now the signal is cut down. With the gain control at the output, turning it down reduces the level of the distorted signal. The distortion is still present, just less intense. If the gain control is placed at the input, the result is that the signal is decreased and becomes closer to the noise level in each stage. There is no distortion, but the noise appears to be greater.

For this reason, in most amplifiers a compromise is reached and the control is placed in the middle of the circuit. This means that the noise from the earlier stages is attenuated and the signal fed to the output is decreased so that there is less likelihood of delivering too much signal to the output, where it would be distorted. This is not always the case, however. In those situations in which noise can be a problem and in which the designer can be certain that the signal will not exceed a given level of distortion, the gain control is placed directly at the output. For example, in audiometers, the attenuator is placed immediately before the headphones. Because the designer has controlled the signal levels in the audiometer so that there is no danger of appreciable distortion, the signal-to-noise improvement inherent in this positioning of the attenuator is used. The only problem associated with this is that the attenuator must be capable of handling the power to be fed to the headphones. Because power is not inconsiderable at 120 dB SPL, attenuators on audiometers have rather heavy wire in them. For this reason it is not common practice to place gain controls at the output of amplifiers driving loudspeakers, as controls that could handle appreciable amounts of signal are large, expensive, and hot to the touch.

One final type of attenuator meets the problem of "where?" by consisting of two attenuators. In the "ganged" arrangement shown in Figure

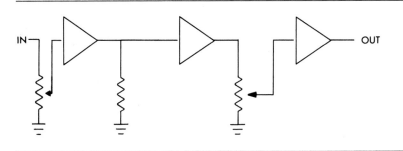

FIG. 3-8.   A circuit with two attenuators.

3-8, both the input and the output are controlled. This connection is common in sound level meters.

Suggested Reading

Beranek, L. L.   *Acoustic Measurements.* New York: Wiley, 1962.

Crowhurst, N. H.   *Basic Audio.* New York: Rider, 1959.

Durrant, J. D., and Lovrinic, J. H.   *Bases of Hearing Science.* Baltimore: Williams & Wilkins, 1984.

Lancaster, D.   *Active Filter Cookbook.* Indianapolis: Sams, 1975.

Malmstadt, H. V., and Enke, C. G.   *Electronics for Scientists.* New York: Benjamin, 1963.

Minifie, F. D., Hixon, T. J., and Williams, F.   *Normal Aspects of Speech, Hearing, and Language.* Englewood Cliffs, N.J.: Prentice-Hall, 1978.

Ryder, J. D.   *Engineering Electronics.* New York: McGraw-Hill, 1957.

Tucker, D. G.   *Elementary Electrical Network Theory.* New York: Macmillan, 1964.

4. Amplifiers

The fundamental building block in almost all electronic equipment today is the amplifier. As the reader achieves a grasp of the theory of amplifier operation he or she can learn to unscramble operating techniques for many unfamiliar pieces of equipment and even devise systems for specific applications. This chapter discusses amplifiers as devices that produce a signal that is a much larger version of the input signal. We also discuss various kinds of signal shaping that can take place in amplifiers without necessarily amplifying the input. Since amplifiers can be arranged to perform various mathematical and electronic operations on input signals and may even decrease their amplitude, we are using the word *amplifier* in its more common usage, which is as a generic term for *signal processor.*

Operating Principles

The amplifier is the heart, in one form or another, of almost every piece of equipment encountered in the audiology laboratory. It is the principal signal processor and may amplify, filter, and modify the input signal in a multitude of ways. The amplifier is such a common and general constituent of electrical systems that it will be discussed in some detail. There is an additional reason for discussing amplifiers: it needs to be made quite clear that the fidelity of a signal can deteriorate inside the electrical domain as well as at the boundary. We must concern ourselves with the fidelity of transduction and transducers but also with the fidelity of transmission and all the components involved. We shall use the discussion of amplifiers to exemplify considerations of signal distortion for a wide variety of equipment.

An amplifier is a device in which an input signal that is typically quite small controls a large source of power (acting like a variable valve), so that the output is an amplified or at least modified version of the input. The important point is that the input signal controls the flow of the power supply, so that the output of the amplifier is a modified image of its small input. We think of an amplifier as being much like the steering mechanism of a power-steering wheel; the more the steering wheel is turned, the more the wheels turn. However, the energy necessary to turn the steering wheel is only a small fraction of the energy necessary to turn the wheels, because the car's power-steering supplies the necessary larger amount of energy that is valved or controlled by the driver's turning of the steering wheel.

There are three parts to the amplifier: power supply, active elements, and controls. The controls, which include on-off switching, overall gain controls or amplification, and tone control (amount of amplification at different frequencies), will be discussed in the following section.

POWER SUPPLY

The *power supply* is a source of DC and consists of batteries or a device that converts the line voltage from a wall plug, which is AC, into a DC of the proper voltage. The size of the power supply plus the efficiency of the amplifier determine the maximum amplification that can be obtained from the amplifier. Because the ultimate output of an amplifier is from this source of power, the power supply will determine the purity or fidelity of the output signal. Often, the distortion from an amplifier is the result of an inadequate power supply.

ACTIVE ELEMENTS

There are two types of *active elements* used in amplifiers: *vacuum tubes* and *solid-state devices*. (Transistors were the first of the solid-state devices that could be used in amplifiers, but there are now many other devices that behave as transistors, and all are grouped under the generic term "solid-state devices.")

For years vacuum tubes served as the active elements in amplifiers, but the invention of the transistor has all but eliminated their use. For information on vacuum-tube operation, see the *Radiotron Designer's Handbook* (listed under Suggested Reading). The transistor was developed at Bell Laboratories where it was discovered that certain materials have the peculiar properties of being neither insulators nor conductors, but semiconductors. Further, if these materials are treated with various impurities, they will have either an excess of negative charges or an excess of holes, which is a lack of negative charges. The former are called N-type materials and the latter P-type materials. If a slice of N-type material is layered with a slice of P-type material, a semiconductor diode will be formed.

Diodes

To understand diode operation, refer to Figure 4-1. The positive charge on the P-type material drives the holes to the junction of the two materials, or *barrier*, because like charges repel and the P-type material is a positive material. The negative pole of the battery drives the electrons in the N-type material to the barrier; if the forces are strong enough, the barrier will be broken down so that current flows across it. (The connection is called *forward-biased*, and the result is a large current flow.) If the battery is connected the other way around, no current flows, because the electrons and holes will be pulled away from the barrier. This latter condition is called *reverse-bias*, and a diode that is reverse-biased will not conduct.

If instead of a battery, a source of AC is connected so that at times the diode is reverse-biased and at other times forward-biased, the resulting current will flow during forward-bias and no current will flow during reverse-bias. Figure 4-2 shows this condition. A sinusoid is applied and the resulting current is a pulsating DC, which is a varying current that never goes negative. The wave is considered to be *half-wave rectified*; the diode is acting as a rectifier. A *rectifier* is any element that changes an AC into a DC. Common rectifiers show a smooth change in current flow when there is a change in applied voltage. The change in current flow is almost linear over a portion of this operating range. In some cases, however, specialized diodes will exhibit other functions. See, for example, the logarithmic function that is used in log operation of operational amplifiers, discussed later.

Semiconductor Amplifiers

To use the transistor as an amplifier, the circuit shown in Figure 4-3 is connected. The P-type material is thin and is sandwiched between two layers of N-type material. If the N-type material is forward-biased with a P-type material, a current will flow (shown at the left of the figure). But the P-type material layer is quite thin, so the electrons travel directly through it to the N-type material, which has a positive charge and attracts electrons. This is the reverse-biased P–N section at the right. The result is current flow. This current flow is a result of the forward bias of one of the P-type materials and the N-type material.

For the purposes of understanding and discussion, we typically describe three aspects or regions of the transistor: the *base, emitter*, and *collector*. The very thin P-type layer is called the base and is the point at

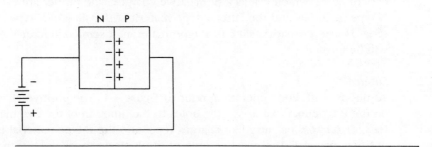

FIG. 4-1.   Semiconductor diode operation.

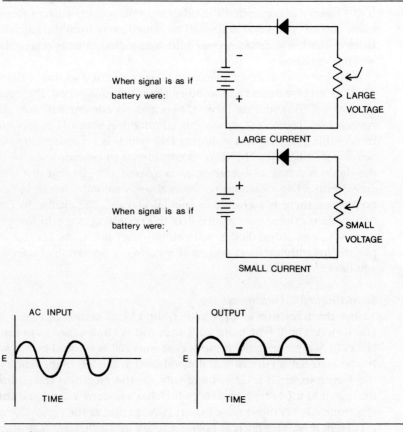

FIG. 4-2.   Diode operation with AC and DC equivalents. E = voltage.

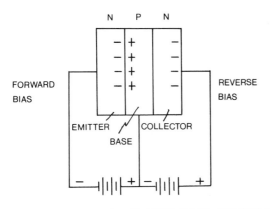

FIG. 4-3. NPN transistor operation.

which the signal is often connected to the amplifier.* The material that
provides the electrons that flow through the circuit is called the emitter,
and the element that accepts the electrons after they flow through the
base is called the collector.

The transistor shown in Figure 4-3 is called an *NPN transistor* because
of the configuration of its layers of materials. It is possible to construct a
PNP transistor, as in Figure 4-4, so that a negative charge on the base
causes it to operate. This is essentially the opposite of the NPN connection. The batteries are reversed from Figure 4-3, but operation is similar
except that current flows in the opposite direction from the NPN transistor.

To examine a transistor operating as an amplifier, consider Figure 4-4,
but replace the forward-bias battery, which is the left-hand one, with a
source of input voltage, such as a microphone. This is shown in Figure
4-5. If the input signal appears as a sine wave, when the sine wave moves
positive, the transistor is forward-biased and conducts. The transistor
conducts at a rate that varies as the input signal varies. However, when
the sine wave moves negative, the transistor is reverse-biased, and the
transistor cannot conduct. Figure 4-6 shows the resultant current associated with input voltage variation. Note that only half the wave is at the
output. To make the amplifier practical for an entire sine wave, the input
is provided with a bias in addition to the input signal. This bias, shown
in Figure 4-7, shifts the forward bias in a positive direction so that it never
goes negative; thus there is always some conduction. Figure 4-8 shows
the resultant input and output waveforms. The input, instead of operating

*There are circuits in which the signal is connected to the emitter or collector, but the
resulting circuit functions in the same way with respect to the biasing of the elements.

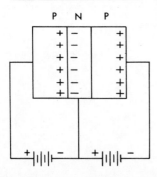

FIG. 4-4.   PNP transistor operation.

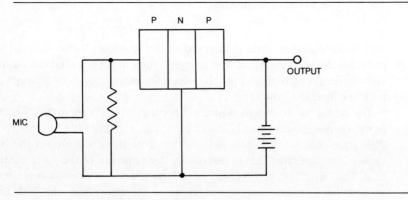

FIG. 4-5.   Single transistor microphone amplifier.

positive and negative around 0 V, operates around the bias value. Now the entire input sine wave is amplified. The permanent forward bias can be supplied by a separate battery or by various types of connections of resistors to the power supply. The multitude of types of bias connectors need not concern us; just remember that a bias should always be present at the input terminal of a transistor for normal amplifier operation. The NPN transistor operates in a similar fashion, but with the polarities reversed, as discussed previously.

Thus far we have talked about a current flowing in the output, but most equipment makes use of voltage variations. To obtain a voltage variation, a resistor (R) is inserted in the output circuit as shown in Figure 4-9. If the current through R varies, the voltage drop across it will vary—Ohm's law once again. Or, if we redraw the situation, we can see that we have a transistor offering a varying amount of resistance to current flow and a fixed resistance in series with it. Figure 4-10 shows just the output

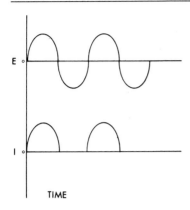

FIG. 4-6.   Input and output waveforms in the circuit shown in Figure 4-5. E = voltage; I = current.

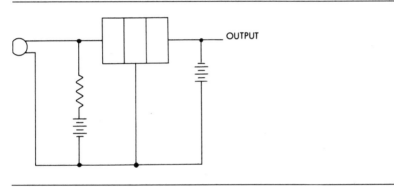

FIG. 4-7.   One method of transistor bias.

circuit. If the transistor resistance decreases (more current flows), more of the power supply voltage (E) will be dropped at R. If the transistor resistance is the same as R, then one-half E will appear across each leg. If the transistor resistance increases (less current flows), more E will appear across the transistor than at R. The result is that the voltage across the transistor varies as a function of the signal, which can then be coupled to later circuits.

In the above discussion, it is apparent that there will always be some voltage across the transistor, even when there is no input signal. In most cases, the AC variation of an input signal is the only output desired. A capacitor is therefore inserted in the output, which effectively eliminates the DC. This circuit is shown in Figure 4-11, where we have the more

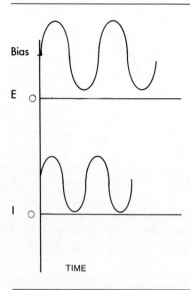

FIG. 4-8.   Input and output waveforms in the circuit shown in Figure 4-7. E = voltage; I = current.

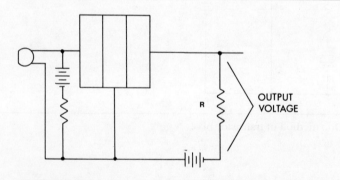

FIG. 4-9.   A circuit with an output resistor (R) to change current variation to voltage variation.

common symbol for the transistor instead of showing the various P and N layers.

Input Impedance

One of the difficulties in designing circuits using transistors is the low impedance that the transistor presents to the device that feeds into it. To clarify this, consider the circuit shown in Figure 4-12.

The generator feeding a signal into the transistor is terminated by the

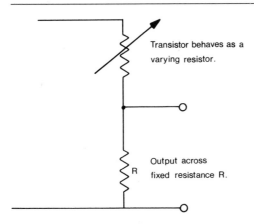

FIG. 4-10. Transistor circuit redrawn with the transistor as a varying resistor (R) and the load as a fixed R.

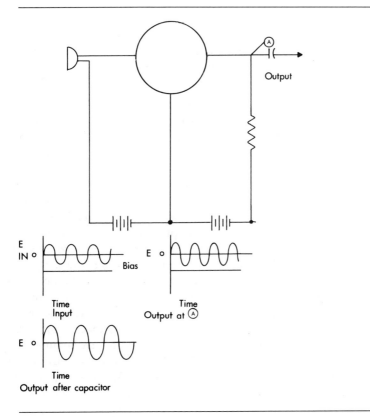

FIG. 4-11. A transistor circuit and the resultant waveforms are shown to demonstrate the effect of a capacitor on the output. E = voltage.

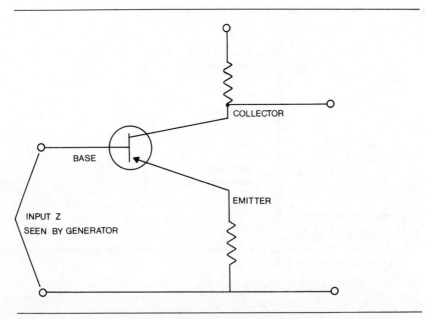

FIG. 4-12.   A transistor circuit and associated impedance seen by a generator feeding the input.

connection between the base and emitter of the transistor. The resistance between these two elements will be small, especially if the device is biased to operate as an amplifier. If the generator is designed to operate into a low resistance, there will be no problem. However, if, for example, electrodes were connected, the electrodes would be essentially shorted because of the small resistance compared to the 5,000- to 100,000-Ω impedance of scalp electrodes. One of the biggest advantages of the vacuum tube is the large resistance it presents to any elements feeding a signal into it. To overcome the low-input impedance problem in many circuits, the input amplifier consists of a device called a *field-effect transistor* (FET). The FET appears as in Figure 4-13. The operating principle may be simplified by saying that current flows through the device until an electrical field is created in the gate. The gate will cause current to decrease by effectively increasing the impedance between source and gate. The FET can be visualized as a pipe whose diameter can be varied by squeezing it. Obviously, if the pipe is squeezed, less liquid can flow. The FET is a conductor surrounded by a material that can cause a field effect, which increases the resistance—the electrical equivalent of squeezing the pipe. The input signal varies the field, which varies the resistance. In the FET, the input is not connected to anything but the gate, which offers a very high impedance. The input, then, is isolated from the remainder of the transistor. The resistance between the gate

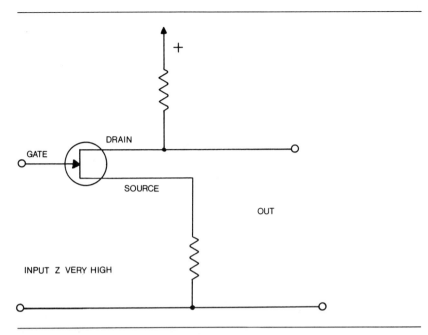

FIG. 4-13.   Field-effect transistor circuit.

and the source is quite large, especially since there is little current flow between the two. For this reason, the generator will see a large impedance. The FET is often used in physiological amplifiers because their input impedance is quite large. Typically, the FET will be followed by the usual solid-state circuits because the output impedance of the FET is small enough to be unaffected by connection to a transistor amplifier.

The active elements in amplifiers have a maximum and minimum output capability, so that if more amplification than is available from one active element is needed, several active elements will be connected serially. Each active element with its associated components is called a *stage*. The signal is connected to the base of a transistor and to ground or the common point of the amplifier.

Active elements in amplifiers are designed to accept signals of various amplitudes and to allow control of various currents. The larger the elements in a vacuum tube or a transistor, the more current it is able to pass. However, large elements in a tube or transistor do not allow precise control of the signal, nor is their sensitivity very high. That is, the input must exceed a specific level before the element will operate. The result of all these conditions is that some tubes and transistors are designed for small input signals and others for large input signals. Amplifiers almost always consist of at least three stages and may have as many as six or seven.

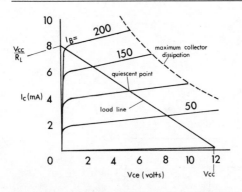

FIG. 4-14. Operating characteristics of ZN94 transistor. R_L = load impedance; Vcc = power supply voltage; I_c = collector current; I_B = base current; Vce = collector-emitter current.

The *dynamic range* of a system is the range, usually expressed in decibels, between the smallest signal that affects the system and the largest signal the system can tolerate. In amplifying systems, the dynamic range may be as small as 10 dB (i.e., the output current can be 3 or more times the input current) and as large as 40 dB (the output current [signal] may be 100 times the input).*

The operation of a transistor circuit is usually plotted on a graph of collecter current versus collecter voltage, with base current as the parameter, called the *operating characteristic curve*. Figure 4-14 shows a set of curves for a common transistor found in many older pieces of equipment. The designer will attempt to operate the device in the linear portion of the characteristic for faithful amplification of the signal. Otherwise, distortion can result. This distortion will be discussed in Chapter 11.

The controls in an amplifier consist of a power switch (on/off switch), a gain control, and, occasionally, tone controls. Different names may be given to the controls, but, in general, the three controls mentioned above are always present in some form or another. There may also be specialized controls for the specific unit. Gain controls and tone controls were discussed previously.

The power switch connects the batteries or the line cord to the amplifier. There may be a lamp associated with the switch so that the user is able to ascertain if the unit is on. If the power switch is a toggle switch, it is conventional that the unit be on when the switch is in the up posi-

*Gain may be calculated using the following formula: Gain (dB) = AV = $20 \log \dfrac{\sqrt{\text{out}}}{\sqrt{\text{in}}}$.

tion and off when down. The switch may also be part of another switch; often it will be connected as part of the gain control, so that if the gain control is rotated full counterclockwise (least gain), the switch clicks off. Another location is on the tone control. In this case it must often be pulled to turn on.

Direct Current Amplifiers

Although most amplifiers in the speech science laboratory are designed to amplify AC signals within the audio range, in some special cases it is desirable to amplify very low frequencies or even DC. For example, in measuring the static pressure within a cavity, the transducer may generate a DC signal proportional to the pressure. If it is necessary to amplify this signal prior to recording, a DC amplifier is required. Suffice it to say that a DC amplifier will amplify *any* voltage change at its input or even within the circuit itself. Because of this ability, if circuit voltages drift or the power supply varies, the result will be a change in the output due to an internal variability. In order to eliminate any drift in the output that is not due to a change at the input, most DC amplifiers have a control labeled either *DC offset* or *DC balance.* To adjust this, the amplifier is connected to an output recording device, such as a voltmeter or scope, with no input signal to the amplifier. If an output is indicated, the balance control is adjusted for zero output. The result is an output free from such internal distortion.

The need to adjust a DC amplifier for drift makes obvious the point that a criterion for selecting DC amplifiers is their stability or freedom from drift. Bear in mind that a DC amplifier will also amplify AC signals, but an AC amplifier can only amplify AC.

There are two general classes of amplifiers, depending on their intended use: voltage amplifiers and power amplifiers.

Voltage Amplifiers

The *voltage amplifier* is used when a signal must be amplified but little or no work is performed. For example, to boost a small electrophysiologic signal to a level for use in an oscilloscope, an increase in voltage is necessary. The oscilloscope operates by moving electrons that are attracted and repelled by an applied voltage and not the amount of current. A voltage amplifier is designed with the assumption that the maximum voltage that the amplifier is capable of handling will be passed through a high impedance. A maximum voltage, determined by the power supply, is delivered across a high impedance:

$$\frac{E}{(\text{large})Z} = (\text{small})\,I$$

where   E = voltage
        Z = impedance
        I = current

Power Amplifiers

But if the work is to be performed there must be both voltage and current; in this case, a *power amplifier* is required. The power amplifier is the device that drives the loudspeaker cone, for example. Here, the designer assumes a maximum voltage across a low impedance. The result of these conditions will be a great deal of current in addition to the maximum voltage: $E/(\text{small})Z = (\text{large})\,I$. The product of voltage times current, expressed in watts, will be a large value of power.

There are other differences between power and voltage amplifiers that we might consider. One is sensitivity; most power amplifiers need about a 1-V input level to provide full power output. Therefore, if a phonograph cartridge is connected to a power amplifier, the result would be very little signal output because the cartridge usually produces a maximum of 10 mV or less. For this reason, a voltage amplifier, called a *preamplifier,* or *preamp* for short, is connected between the cartridge and the power amplifier. The voltage amplifier will step up the 10 mV to 1 to 2 V, which is more than adequate for driving the power amplifier.

Another basic difference is that power amplifiers do not usually have any controls other than a gain control. In the case of music systems, the preamplifier has all the controls, although most music systems today have the preamplifier and power amplifier built on one chassis. In the case of electrophysiological recording systems, the preamplifier may contain filters and gain controls; its power amplifier usually has only a gain control.

Often, for both research and home listening purposes, amplification equipment is designed so that low-level amplifiers (or preamplifiers) are separated from high signal-level power amplifiers. In general, this design decision comes out of considering the signal conditions themselves. In a preamplifier, signal levels (variations in signal voltage) are very small and are amplified significantly prior to final transduction; often amplification by factors of 1,000 to 1 (60 dB) or 10,000 to 1 (80 dB) occurs in a combination of preamplifier and amplifier. Not only will the signal be amplified greatly, but any distortion in the signal will be equally amplified. More to the point, because the signal to be amplified is of such low level, even a small amount of distortion can easily be as large as the signal itself. Therefore, maintaining signal quality and an appropriately low level of distortion places great demands on all components and particularly on the purity of the output of the power supply.

The power supply is the source of the even or constant flow of electrons through the circuit; this flow is modulated by the signal variations, so that the output is an enlarged representation of the input. It is the power supply that is the source for the increase in power. The signal itself acts to "valve" the power supply so as to achieve amplification with minimal distortion.

In contrast to a preamplifier, the power supply of an amplifier need not be so stringently designed because any distortion it may introduce into the signal will be a small part of the signal energy (the signal itself already having undergone significant amplification in the preamplifier).

Any controls to be introduced into the circuit—filtering, equalization, overall gain, balancing channels, or whatever—are most often introduced into the preamplifier where signal levels are low and power supplies are more stringently designed. With controls in the preamplifier, more sensitive and more distortion-free control can be attained. That is, the control components can then be built to handle only low power levels and the designer has better controlled power supplies if the design requires them.

The last differences of importance are the physical size and heat. The voltage amplifier is smaller than the power amplifier and does not generate any appreciable amount of heat. The power amplifier is large, heavy, and must be provided with adequate air circulation around it because it is generating power, not all of which is available for work; much is simply wasted in the form of heat.

Most solid-state power amplifiers have the output transistors mounted on finned aluminum brackets for the purpose of carrying away the heat. They may even have fans. The operator should make certain that there is adequate air circulation around any power amplifiers, especially solid-state units. Excessive heat readily destroys transistors.

In almost all cases, it is possible to short the two input leads of any amplifier together without damage to the amplifier. This is a part of the method of measuring signal-to-noise ratio. However, the output connections should never be shorted together. Almost all solid-state equipment manufactured today has provisions for temporary *overload,* which is what happens when the output is shorted. If a short occurs, elements sense that a great deal more current than is proper is flowing or that the unit is heating up, and the power supply shuts itself off until the problem is corrected. In spite of this, never take the chance of shorting the output.

Operational Amplifiers

A general class of amplifiers that has found wide usage in the clinic and laboratory in the past few years is the operational amplifier, or op amp for short. These are general purpose devices whose processing abilities

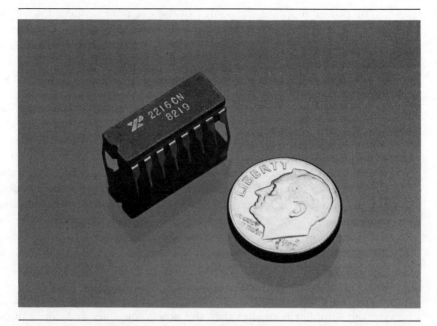

FIG. 4-15.   Integrated circuit containing operational amplifiers. (Courtesy Exar
Corporation, Sunnyvale, CA.)

can be manipulated by varying external components attached to them.
To explain further, the operational amplifier is an amplifier with extremely high gain. (In most computations the gain is assumed to be infinite, but most operational amplifiers have gains of 1,000 to 100,000.)

The usual operational amplifier is small, as can be seen from Figure 4-
15. It is an off-the-shelf tool and can be applied to almost any system in
which gain or signal generation or conditioning is necessary. Usually a
single integrated circuit (IC) chip will contain two to six operational
amplifiers.

The operational amplifier has two inputs, one labeled + and the other
labeled −. These indicate that the plus input will cause an output in
phase with the input signal, while the minus will cause an output 180°
out of phase with the input. The latter is called the *inverter input.*

The secret of the operational amplifier is feedback. That is, some of
the output is fed back to the input through various configurations of
external components. The input to the amplifier is through an electronic
component that, in conjunction with the feedback components, determines the gain and transfer function of the operational amplifier.

To operate the amplifier as a simple amplifying device, the signal is fed
in through a resistor and the feedback is through a resistor. The gain of
the amplifier is the ratio of the two resistors. Examine Figure 4-16. The

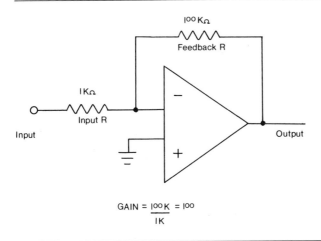

$$GAIN = \frac{100 \text{ K}}{1 \text{ K}} = 100$$

FIG. 4-16.   Operational amplifier gain computation. R = resistor.

gain of the amplifier shown is 100, because the ratio of feedback to input is 100 to 1. The feedback need not be in the form of a resistor, however. If other elements are used, the amplifier will generate various mathematical functions. A more complete discussion of operational amplifiers will be found in Chapter 14.

There are situations in which one wishes to sum a continuous voltage over a period of time. For example, if an assessment of total amount of air exhaled over the length of an utterance is the measure of interest, the output of a pneumotachograph that measures volume velocity can be utilized. The *integrator* is a device that sums the input over a period of time, determined by the operator or by the limits of the machine. Figure 4-17 shows an integrator. The switch (SW) functions to discharge the capacitor so that another integration can begin. Thus, the electrical signal proportional to the volume velocity is summed over a period of time. The sum equals the total air expelled (the exhaled volume), for example. If a timer controls a relay placed across the capacitor, the integration will take place for the duration of the timer's interval.

When the capacitor is moved to the input the result is a *differentiator*. The differentiator gives an output that is proportional to *the change* in the input signal. The change in signal is analogous to acceleration, which is a change in velocity. If the velocity were constant, there would be no acceleration and no change in signal and, therefore, no output from the differentiator. That is, if a signal has a constant value, there would be no output, but if the signal were turned off suddenly, the output would jump to a high negative value because the input changed abruptly. The value would return to zero quickly if the signal stayed off, but jump to a posi-

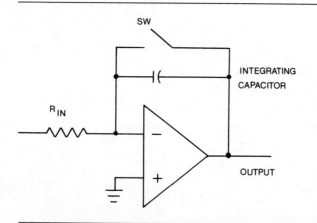

FIG. 4-17.   Integrator circuit. SW = switch; R_{IN} = input resistor.

tive value if the signal were restarted. That is, the differentiator gives an output that is proportional to velocity, if the input represents displacement. Were a square wave to be fed into a differentiator, the output would be as in Figure 4-18. Notice that an output occurs only when the square wave changes its amplitude.

It should be apparent from these few examples that the operational amplifier can perform many functions, dependent upon external connections to the various inputs and outputs on the amplifier. This ability is what makes the operational amplifier the instrument of choice in a majority of laboratory systems. Several more examples will further illustrate the flexibility of the amplifier.

To sum several voltages (or, with any slight changes, currents), several input resistors are added. As before, the gain of the amplifier is equal to the ratio of R_{out}/R_{in}. If all the input resistors are 10,000 Ω and the feedback resistor is 100,000 Ω, the gain is equal to 10 for all inputs. But the output will be a composite signal of all the inputs, with equal gain. Of course, the input resistor values could be juggled to obtain differing amounts of gain for each of the inputs. Such a circuit, as in Figure 4-19, is called a *summer circuit*, which is a type of *mixer;* that is, it mixes several inputs into one output (as discussed in the following section, Mixers).

To construct a *subtracter,* one input is connected to the + terminal and the other to the − . The result is an output that is the sum of "plus" one signal and "minus" the other. Several signals may be summed and subtracted from several other signals, as in Figure 4-20.

The main advantage and application of operational amplifiers is the fact that they are small, inexpensive, general-purpose devices that can be operated for many purposes with many different characteristics by chang-

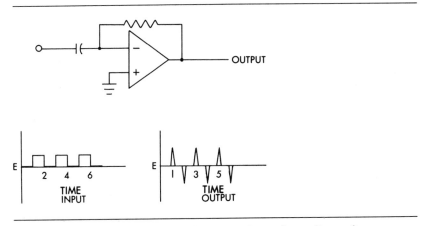

FIG. 4-18.   Differentiator circuit and associated waveforms. E = voltage.

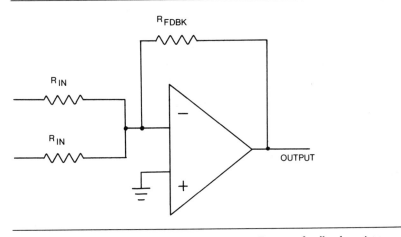

FIG. 4-19.   Summer circuit. R_{IN} = input resistor; R_{FDBK} = feedback resistor.

ing only a few external components. There is no necessity to change the
design of the amplifier. The flexibility of the operational amplifier can be
illustrated by the fact that a given unit can be used as a physiological
amplifier by connecting skin electrodes to the plus and minus input terminals, which results in cancellation of any noise current induced in the
electrode wires by stray fields and varying the gain by changing feedback
resistors. Note that the cancellation occurs because the output is the sum
of the amplified signals at + and − inputs, but the output due to the +
is in phase with the input, and the output at the − is 180° out of phase,
as in Figure 4-21. If the output is the sum of these, the result is the ad-

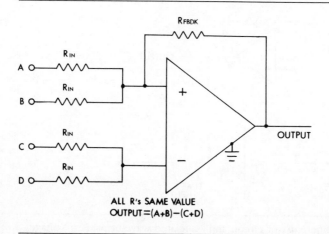

FIG. 4-20.   Summer/subtracter circuit. R_{IN} = input resistor; R_{FDBK} = feedback resistor.

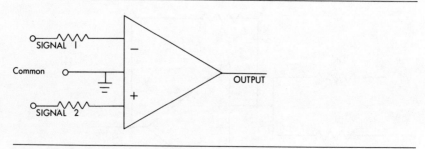

FIG. 4-21.   Differential amplifier circuit.

dition of two signals exactly 180° out of phase. Thus, if any noise voltage has been induced in the electrode wires, the noise voltage will be cancelled. But because the two electrodes are at different places, the two *signals* will probably not be in phase, so they will not cancel but be amplified, and the output will be the sum of both inputs being amplified. This operation is called *differential amplification* and is almost always used in electrophysiologic recording.

To show how amplifier theory can be applied, we will consider airflow measurement. If we are interested in the rate of flow, we would use only an amplifier connected to the transducer, but if we wanted *total airflow,* we would use an integrator. If we were interested only in change of flow, as when evaluating dysfluency, we might use a differentiator, which would give a signal proportional to change in flow rate. And if we were interested in a value proportional to the ratio of nasal-to-oral airflow, we might connect two transducers, one to the mouth and one to the nose, and feed the signals to a subtracter. The output would be proportional to the amount of oral airflow in excess of the amount of nasal airflow.

Mixers

In some cases it may be desirable to mix two signals, as, for example, when recording the narration during a therapy session. This is a simple operation as long as the impedance seen by the inputs and sources are proper. Consider connecting two 50-Ω microphones. Each microphone would "see" the impedance of the other and be effectively short-circuited. To avoid this, a mixer is used, containing preamplifiers that boost each input and then mix the signals. Figure 4-22 illustrates the technique. The output impedance of each amplifier is sufficiently small that it is not disturbed by being connected to the other amplifier. Similarly, the inputs are isolated by the amplifiers. The technique can be used for more than two inputs by simply adding amplifiers. Operational amplifiers are often used for this mixing.

To feed one output to several inputs, called *fanout,* the output device can be simply hooked to multiple cables, provided the output impedance is low enough. Again, an operational amplifier can be used; it will have

FIG. 4-22.   Microphone mixer circuit. R_{IN} = input resistor; R_{FDBK} = feedback resistor.

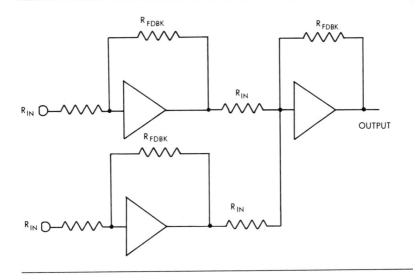

an output impedance of only a few ohms. The only caveat in fanout is to avoid ground loops by making certain that there is only one good solid ground side to the connections.

Summary

This chapter, like the initial chapter, has covered a large amount of ground (no pun intended). Amplifiers are at the heart of most pieces of electronic equipment, and they are important even though they are conceptually simple. Each consists of a power supply, active elements, and some controls. The amplifier accepts an input and enlarges or amplifies it. The amplifier must be constructed so that it can handle, with appropriate fidelity, both the amplitude range desired (i.e., the input has to be sufficiently strong that the internal noise does not cause it to deteriorate by more than some minimal amount, but not so strong that it exceeds the limits of the amplifier components, which would result in distorting the signal) and the frequency passband desired (otherwise the amplifier acts as a filter).

The amplifier works by using the input signal to control or valve the power supply so that the signal at the amplifier output is an amplified version of its input. Note, however, that amplifiers may also serve as the active elements in filters, circuits to perform mathematical functions, and instruments to isolate parts of an equipment array.

Suggested Reading

Crowhurst, N. H.   *Basic Audio.* New York: Rider, 1959.

Langford-Smith, F.   *Radiotron Designer's Handbook.* Harrison, N. J.: RCA, 1957.

Malmstadt, H. V., and Enke, C. G.   *Electronics for Scientists.* New York: Benjamin, 1963.

Malmstadt, H. V., and Enke, C. G.   *Digital Electronics for Scientists.* New York: Benjamin, 1969.

Minifie, F. D., Hixon, T. J., and Williams, F.   *Normal Aspects of Speech, Hearing, and Language.* Englewood Cliffs, N.J.: Prentice-Hall, 1978.

Ryder, J. D.   *Engineering Electronics.* New York: McGraw-Hill, 1957.

5. Transformers

We have chosen to discuss transformers in a separate chapter because transformers fulfill rather specific needs without relating to other devices very readily. Transformers are devices that can isolate parts of a circuit, raise or lower voltages, and match impedances. For example, if we place a secondary coil of a material with magnetic properties within the magnetic field of a primary coil and introduce some kind of varying electrical signal to the primary coil, it will induce a voltage into the secondary. The voltage in the secondary coil will vary with the varying signal voltage. The result of this magnetic "coupling" is that a signal can be passed from one coil to another, even though the circuits containing the coils remain independent of one another. The impedance of each coil is determined by the number of turns in the coil and some characteristics of the wire in it (e.g., diameter, composition). Finally, as we shall see, the voltage amplitude in the secondary coil is related to the voltage amplitude in the primary coil as well as to the number of turns in each coil. Each of these characteristics is put to use in different transformer applications: for example, they can be used to step up or step down voltage, to obtain a particular impedance in a primary or a secondary coil or both, to isolate two circuits from one another, and so on.

Essentially, a transformer consists of a core of iron alloy around which is wrapped two or more coils as shown in Figure 5-1. When a voltage is connected to one coil (called the *primary*), magnetic lines of force will induce an electromagnetic field (EMF) in the other coils (called the *secondaries*). It is possible to have more than one primary coil and more than one secondary.

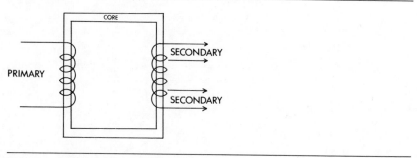

FIG. 5-1.   Schematic of a transformer.

Voltage Change

The efficiency of a transformer is nearly 100%. Therefore, if there are twice as many turns in the secondary as the primary, the voltage in the secondary will be twice that of the primary. The law of conservation of energy says that the power in the two sides of the transformer must be equal, so if the secondary voltage is doubled, the current must be halved. You cannot deliver more energy than that which is provided to the primary. This is analogous to a lever. If you push on the longer arm of the lever it must move a greater distance than the shorter arm. However, the force exerted by the shorter arm will be greater and its movement restricted, so that the work done—force × distance—is equal in each arm. The result of transformer action, then, is that $E_p I_p = E_s I_s$. The product of the voltage in the primary (E_p) times current in the primary (I_p) (the power in the primary) is equal to the product of the voltage in the secondary (E_s) times current in the secondary (I_s). If voltage is stepped up, current will be proportionally stepped down, and vice versa; one use of a transformer is to alter voltage level or magnitude systematically.

Impedance Change

Another use of a transformer is to alter the impedance of a device in a circuit. The coil of wire in the primary exhibits some impedance, which is partially a function of the number of turns in the coil and partially a function of the diameter of the wire, the diameter of the coil, the form on which the coil is wound, and other factors. If the secondary has more turns than the primary, the impedance of the secondary will be increased in comparison to the primary. The relationship that holds here is: $Z_s = Z_p (N_s/N_p)^2$. The impedance of the secondary (Z_s) is equal to the impedance of the primary (Z_p) multiplied by the turns ratio squared. The *turns ratio* is the number of turns in the secondary (N_s) divided into the number of turns in the primary (N_p). For example, to construct a power supply providing 40 V, but which plugs into a wall outlet, we need to step down from the 110 V supplied by the power company to the 40 V we require. A transformer having 2.75 more turns on the primary than on the secondary would provide this step-down effect. Let us think about why the turns ratio must be 2.75 turns on the primary coil for each turn of the secondary coil. First, the greater the number of turns, the higher the impedance; the higher the impedance, the greater the voltage drop. As previously stated, the voltage ratio is determined by the turns ratio. If we are to have a voltage drop of 110 V in the primary but only 40 V in the secondary, then there must be more windings in the primary. The ratio of the windings is the same as the ratio of the two voltage drops, which is $110/40 = 2.75$.

As another and common example, if your pocket calculator works by either a 9-V battery or by plugging it into the wall outlet, then the calculator incorporates a transformer. The transformer, typically a bulbous portion of the power cord, must reduce the 110 V from the power company to 9 V. The voltage ratio of 110 V/9 V is 12.222, so that the transformer primary coil must have 12.222 windings for each winding of the secondary. There are some modern electrical circuits that perform the transformer function of stepping voltage up or down, but they are sufficiently rare that we need not concern ourselves with them.

Isolation

Still another use of a transformer is for isolation. At times we may wish to isolate a piece of equipment from the earth ground provided by the power lines (see the discussion of Ground in Chap. 1). This isolation can be provided by connecting the equipment to the power lines through a transformer having a turns ratio of 1. Thus there will be 110 V on both primary and secondary, but neither side of the secondary needs to be connected to the ground. The isolation transformer is commonly used to isolate from the power line inexpensive equipment that has been designed without a power transformer. The power transformer can isolate the equipment from ground, but a manufacturer can save money by eliminating it.

Impedance-matching

A transformer may be used to match impedances. A low impedance microphone can be connected to an instrument that normally is connected to a high-impedance device. This is accomplished by means of a transformer whose primary matches the impedance of the microphone and whose secondary matches the input impedance of the instrument. For example, to connect a 500-Ω microphone to an amplifier that is designed to "see" an input Z of 10,000 Ω, a transformer could be used with a 500-Ω primary and a turns ratio of 4.47. To understand the necessity for a turns ratio of 4.47, let us take time to do the calculation. We earlier stated the relationship between primary and secondary impedances and turns as $Z_s = Z_p (N_s/N_p)^2$. The impedance ratio of secondary to primary is the square root of the turns ratio of secondary to primary. In our example, the impedance ratio is 10,000 to 500, or 20 to 1. Therefore, the turns ratio of secondary to primary when squared must be 20 to 1; that is, the turns ratio per se must be the square root of 20, which is 4.47. A special transformer is used when connecting balanced microphones to many amplifiers, as described in Chapter 6.

This book does not discuss power supplies in any detail, but power transformers are commonly used in power supplies to step the line voltage of 110 V or 220 V up or down for the operation of vacuum tubes or solid-state devices.

III. Generation, Storage, and Measurement of Signals

6. Transducers

This chapter on transducers is incomplete, because Chapters 8, 9, and 12 also deal with transducers. In this chapter, we consider mostly microphones and loudspeakers, that is, the transducers into and out of the acoustic domain, plus some few other transducers that will help in generalizing the principles.

The transducer is a device that converts one form of energy to another. It may consist of a microphone, loudspeaker, or, for example, a light bulb. This chapter discusses most of the common types of transducers found in the laboratory and the clinic, but there is such a proliferation of these devices that the chapter cannot be considered comprehensive. Also, it is often possible that a transducer designed for one application can be modified to fulfill the requirements of another. For example, how might the shiver of an animal be measured in a behavioral modification program? The animal is presented with a tone and then a blast of cold air. The stimuli are paired in this way until the animal shivers each time the tone is presented, whether a blast of cold air follows it or not. How might the shiver be measured? The animal can be placed on a spring-mounted platform with stereo phonograph cartridges underneath. The styli barely touch the underside of the platform. If the platform moves, the styli move and an output that is equivalent to the movement of the platform is generated. The interested student will probably see many other situations in which different systems might be utilized in measuring disparate dimensions.

As our introduction to transducers, consider first the microphone, the most common transducer.

Input Transducers

MICROPHONES

A microphone is a device that causes an electrical current to flow as a function of a changing acoustic signal at the face of the microphone. Most microphones respond to a changing sound pressure, but this is not always the case, as the student will note in the following discussion.

Dynamic Microphones

One of the least expensive and most popular microphones is called the *dynamic.* It consists of a coil of wire attached to a paper cone. The coil surrounds a permanent magnet. If the coil is moved, a current will be induced as a function of the lines of force of the magnet cut by the moving coil. The cone-coil combination is suspended at the edges and is free to move as the sound strikes the cone. Figure 6-1 illustrates this type of microphone.

Crystal Microphones

The crystal microphone is also one of the least expensive to construct and, in the past, was usually the type found with inexpensive tape recorders. It consists of a slab of crystal (any one of several different kinds) connected to the case of the microphone at one end and at the other to the cone or diaphragm of the microphone. When sound strikes the cone, the crystal is bent, which results in a current. The phenomenon of a crystal generating a current when it is bent is called the *piezoelectric effect.* Figure 6-2 shows a crystal microphone.

Condenser Microphones

Because of its broad frequency response, the condenser microphone is typically the microphone of choice for precision measurements, such as audiometer calibration. This microphone uses the principle of a capacitor to operate. (*Condenser* is another name for capacitors, but it is an obsolete term except in the description of microphones.) Figure 6-3 shows a circuit with a large value of resistor, a power supply, and a capacitor. The power supply charges the capacitor to a value that is partially determined by the size of the capacitor and partially by the spacing of the two plates. If anything, such as acoustic pressure, alters this spacing, the charge on the capacitor will vary. This variation in charge causes a current to flow as the capacitor charges to different values. The result is a current flow through the large resistor, which causes a voltage to appear across the large resistor. This voltage is proportional to the variation in the charge on the capacitor, which, in turn, is a function of the spacing of the plates.

Figure 6-4 illustrates a microphone using this principle. A very thin and light plate of metal is placed above another plate isolated from the

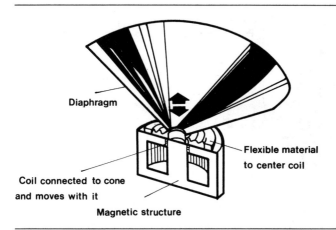

FIG. 6-1. General construction of a dynamic microphone.

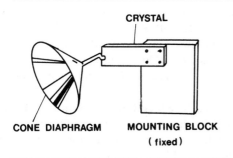

FIG. 6-2. General construction of a crystal microphone.

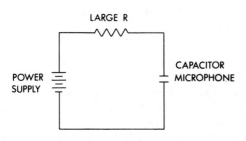

FIG. 6-3. General schematic of a condenser (capacitor) microphone. R = resistor.

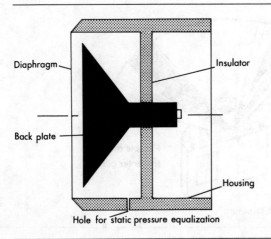

Diaphragm

Insulator

Back plate

Housing

Hole for static pressure equalization

FIG. 6-4.   Schematic construction of a condenser microphone.

housing. The two plates are isolated from one another and thus form a capacitor. If the unit is placed in the circuit of Figure 6-3 and varying sound pressure causes the thin plate to flex, a varying electrical current equivalent to the changing sound pressure will result. The only moving element in this microphone is the very thin diaphragm, so its frequency response is quite broad. Figure 6-5 illustrates a modern condenser microphone.

The condenser microphone is a very high impedance device. Because of its extreme lack of sensitivity it will usually have a very small amplifier and impedance-matching circuit built into the case along with the microphone. The output impedance of this is quite small, and the resulting output is the same as if a low-impedance microphone were used.

Electret Microphones
The electret microphone is a recently invented microphone that behaves in much the same manner as the condenser microphone but has a permanent charge on it, thereby eliminating the external power supply. It is inexpensive but can be of high quality relative to other types of inexpensive microphones.

Considerations in Microphone Use
There are several points that bear consideration in using microphones and in obtaining the best possible results with them.

First of all, *do not place the microphone too close to the mouth.* Some speech sounds, especially the plosives, are accompanied by a blast of air that may cause the microphone to be driven beyond its limits and cause it to produce a signal that is not really part of the pattern of the phoneme.

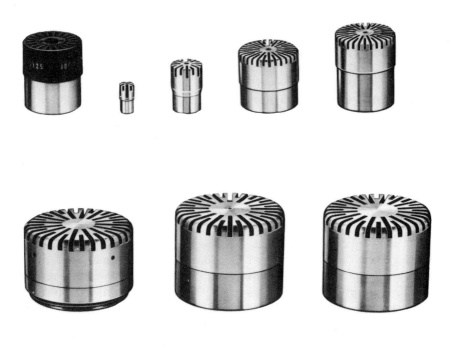

FIG. 6-5. Modern condenser microphones for various applications. (Courtesy Bruel & Kjaer Instruments, Inc., Cleveland, OH.)

The result is a terrible "pop" or, worse, overdriving of the unit to which the signal is fed, and sometimes even blocking. *Blocking* is a phenomenon in which an amplifier ceases working for a brief period of time because of an overload. Some microphones have acoustic filters across the diaphragm to prevent some of this blast, but filters may influence the frequency response and sensitivity of the microphone. (An acoustic filter can be something as simple as a layer or two of gauze-like material.)

Avoid physical abuse of the microphone. Condenser and crystal microphones are especially fragile. When using a microphone, do not hold it by its cord; such handling weakens connections. Avoid dropping a microphone, as there are elements inside that can be knocked out of alignment. For example, if the coil in a dynamic microphone is knocked askew, the output may be very distorted.

Do not expose the microphone to high temperatures or humidity. Condenser microphones are especially prone to damage from high humidity. If moisture condenses between the plates, it can cause a short circuit that may burn the plates or destroy the preamplifier. It is best to store condenser microphones with a dessicant (drying agent), which is usually supplied with the microphone.

Always use a microphone stand when possible. Microphones generate a voltage no matter what causes the diaphragm to move. Holding the microphone in the hand may cause enough jiggling to generate an unwanted signal. If a table stand is used to support the microphone, be sure that the table is sturdy. A flimsy table may cause vibration of the unit and another unwanted signal. Also, try to keep from disturbing the cord, which may cause noise by transmitting vibrations to the microphone. If using a lavaliere microphone, which hangs by a cord around the neck, be sure to use a clip to fasten the cord so that it does not rub.

Impedance is an important characteristic in the selection and use of a microphone, particularly if the microphone is to be connected by a very long cable. The reasons for considering the relationship between impedance and cable length is that there are a variety of varying magnetic (electrical) fields in most locations. These fields may arise from light bulbs, nearby radio stations, other electronic equipment, power lines, or whatever. If the cable connecting the microphone to an amplifier is sufficiently close to such varying fields, the varying magnetism will introduce some small electrical flow (current) in the microphone cable.

Consider the situation with a crystal microphone, which is a high impedance device. The nearby magnetic fields introduce a variety of noises; the significant noise current will cause the signal to deteriorate because of the high impedance. That is, some small current in combination with a high resistance results in a large voltage.

The situation with a dynamic microphone, whch is a low-impedance device, is quite different. Assuming the same magnetic fields, we must contend with the same noise current, but that same noise current flowing through a low impedance is a small voltage, and the signal-to-noise ratio will still be acceptable.

The problem with high impedance microphones is that any small current, such as might be picked up in the microphone cable from a nearby stray electromagnetic field, will generate a voltage that might approach the magnitude of the signal generated by the microphone. Therefore, a low-impedance microphone should always be used if possible, and microphone cords should be kept as short as possible.

In situations where there is a great deal of electromagnetic radiation or where long cords are used, one may choose the special tactic of using a balanced microphone system in combination with a coaxial cable. A *coaxial cable* is one in which the conductors within the cable are enveloped within a metallic shield, which acts as a third conductor.

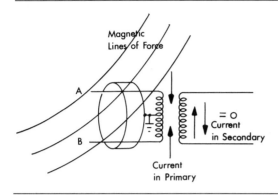

FIG. 6-6.   Induced current in cable and transformer of a balanced microphone.

Figure 6-6 shows a circuit used when electromagnetic radiation is quite large. All of the conductors are connected to a transformer. If electromagnetic lines of force from electrically noisy devices induce a current in the conductors, the current will flow in the same direction for all three conductors. The braided shield (represented by the rings around the input wires), however, surrounds the other two wires and is connected directly to ground. Thus, if a current is induced in it, it will be shunted directly to ground. It is possible that some of the lines of force may leak through the braided shield and induce a current in the other two conductors. The current flow is in the same direction in both wires. Wire A and ground allow a current in the direction of the top arrow. Wire B and ground also allow a current in the direction of the bottom arrow. A current is induced in the secondary by both these primaries, but the currents are in opposite directions, so the result is no current in the secondary if the two primaries are matched and balanced. The result is complete cancellation of all the induced noise.

To connect a microphone to the arrangement discussed above, it is necessary to have a microphone with two coils attached to the diaphragm. When the diaphragm moves, currents are induced in the two microphone coils and, in turn, in the two transformer primary coils. The currents are out of phase with respect to ground but in phase with respect to the secondary coil, as shown in Figure 6-7. The result is a current induced in the secondary by each of the primaries, but because they are in phase with respect to the secondary, there is no cancellation, and all the primary current is coupled to the secondary. The secondary of the transformer can then be connected to any amplifier. The microphone and transformer arrangement described above is called a *balanced microphone* and is always used in environments in which a great deal of electromagnetic radiation might be present and in cases where very long microphone cables are necessary (100–500 feet).

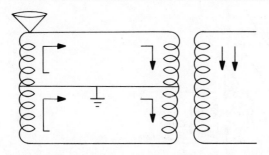

FIG. 6-7. Signal current in microphone coil, cable, and transformer of a balanced microphone.

PHONOGRAPH CARTRIDGES

Other types of input transducers may be encountered in the laboratory. Phonograph cartridges are probably the input transducers with which people are most familiar, inasmuch as they are encountered in every home. Most cartridges consist of a pair of coils connected to the stylus, which rides in the record grooves. The coils are placed near permanent magnets; as the stylus is wiggled by the record grooves, the coils are wiggled near the magnets and a current is induced. Two coils are necessary for the two channels in stereo recordings.

ACCELEROMETERS

The accelerometer is another useful input transducer that is finding its way into the speech science area. Figure 6-8 shows the principal parts of the device. Note that it consists of a mass suspended and shaped to enclose a permanent magnet. A coil is attached to the mass and wraps around the magnet. When the accelerometer case moves, the mass suspended by the spring will move, but with a slight delay because of its inertia. The coil reflects the movement of the mass to which it is attached; because the coil is moving relative to the magnet, a current is induced in it. Leads (wires) from the coil carry the induced current to a following amplifier circuit. Figure 6-9 illustrates a commercially available accelerometer.

The accelerometer is attached to an object whose acceleration is to be measured. For example, it might be glued to the mandible. When the mandible moves, the accelerometer case moves, but the mass lags slightly behind because of inertia. The magnets attached to the case move with respect to the coil attached to the mass. The result is a current proportional to the acceleration of the object. Accelerometers are low-impedance devices and in other respects operate as microphones.

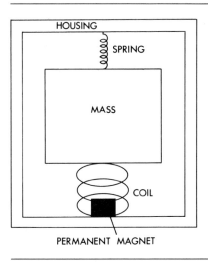

FIG. 6-8. Schematic of the construction of an accelerometer.

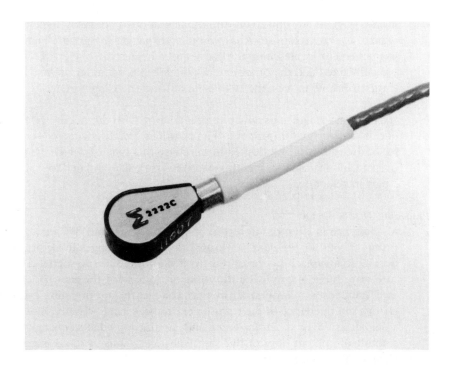

FIG. 6-9. A microminiature accelerometer measuring about 1 × ½ cm.

STRAIN GAUGES

Strain gauges are simply tiny sheets of material that can be glued to objects and generate a current as a result of the piezoelectric effect or change their resistance when bent. Thus, they will generate a current as a function of the distortion of the surface on which they are glued or their resistance will vary, which can result in a varying current if they are connected to a source of voltage. They have been glued to the soft palate, for example. When the soft palate is moved during speech, a current is recorded that relates to the closure of the velopharyngeal mechanism. Strain gauges are high-impedance devices and must have short leads to them. They come in a variety of sizes, but the ones most often used in the speech science labs are quite small—about ½ × ½ inch. To attach the gauge to some external apparatus, the wires are usually microwelded in place. Heat used in soldering may damage the elements. Also, the wires are so small that any other type of attachment except welding is often unsuccessful, although some experts have been soldering them for years. To attach the gauge to the surface whose deformation is being measured, a special adhesive supplied by the gauge manufacturer is used.

Often, two gauges are used in order to increase the sensitivity. A gauge is placed on either side of a piece of metal to assess its bend; for example, if one gauge bends concavely, the other will bend convexly. As a matter of fact, several investigators have used strain gauges to measure mandibular movement by attaching the gauges to a metal strip, one end of which is rigidly fixed and the other end of which is placed under the mandible. If the mandible moves, the strip is flexed and the gauges generate a signal.

The strain gauge is usually purchased along with the necessary amplifier, since the input impedance of an amplifier greatly affects the sensitivity of the gauge. If one desires to purchase this type of device, its sensitivity (which is usually directly related to size), size, and material all play a part in selection.

PRESSURE TRANSDUCERS

Air pressure is often of interest in assessing normal and deviant speech. Instantaneous air pressure, static air pressure, or changes in air pressure over time may each be measured. To make these measurements, a pressure transducer is employed. It works on somewhat the same principle as a condenser microphone, in that changes in air pressure cause a change in impedance of the transducer. In measuring pressure, however, a signal is fed to the transducer and, as the impedance changes, the amount of current flow of the signal changes. Thus, if there is a static change in pressure, the current flow is constant, but at some value other than zero. This is not the case in microphones, where an output occurs

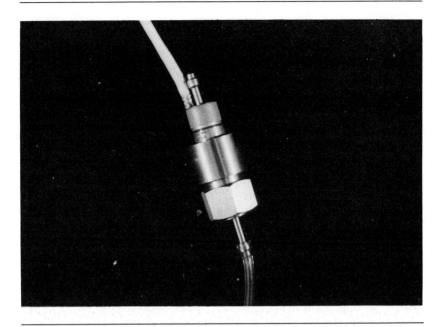

FIG. 6-10.   A pressure transducer of the kind used in measuring intraoral air pressure (60 mm in length × 22 mm in diameter).

only as a result of some change. Figure 6-10 shows one type of pressure transducer.

Output Transducers

LOUDSPEAKERS

Output transducers work on the same principles as the input transducers that have been discussed. A coil is attached to a cone of paper and wrapped around one end of a magnetic rod (see Fig. 6-1). When a current is applied to the coil, the magnet alternately attracts and repels the coil (depending on the direction of the current flow), causing the cone of paper to move.

An alternative to the permanent magnet speaker is the electrostatic speaker. The electrostatic speaker is constructed of a large sheet of material—typically plastic film—on which an electrostatic charge is placed. The material is then attracted to or reflected from its metal frame because of a varying voltage (the signal) delivered to the metal. The large moving surface of the material moves air particles because of its own movement, thereby transducing the voltage to a pressure wave in air.

Speakers tend to be large because they must move a sufficient number of air particles to generate appropriately loud sound in the space in which they operate. Most loudspeakers are 8 to 12 inches in diameter, although there are speakers smaller than 1 inch and as large as 30 inches. Most headphones, having to operate into the space of an ear canal, are simply very small speakers. One common exception to this rule are crystal headphones, which are discussed in a following section.

A condenser microphone or any other microphone could be used as an output transducer, at least in theory. Many practical problems prevent such use except in rare instances, but the ideas are worth our consideration. A most important consideration is that the plate of any microphone receiving pressure variation is typically quite small so that it will be moved easily by variations in air pressure. A loudspeaker, on the other hand, must move relatively large quantities of air to create sound pressure of sufficient level to be heard at a reasonable distance. An additional consideration is that a speaker is constructed of material that has very different properties from the medium in which it operates so that there is typically a large impedance mismatch to overcome, resulting in much energy wastage.

The loudspeaker operating into a medium will move air in front of the cone but behind it also; that is, it puts out a front wave and a back wave. As the back wave travels around the speaker to go forward, it effectively creates an echo to the front wave, so that a speaker must be enclosed in order not to distort its own output. There are two opposite ways of dealing with the back wave. The first is to suppress it by using an acoustic absorbing material to line or to fill the interior of the speaker enclosure. The second is to time the enclosure; that is, to make it an acoustic resonating chamber so as to enhance the sound reproduction of the speaker. High fidelity loudspeakers come in both varieties, with some discerning listeners preferring one, some preferring the other. Figure 6-11 shows the construction of a permanent magnet loudspeaker.

When a current is fed into the coil, the coil is alternately attracted and repelled by the magnet, and it moves. The coil is attached to a cone of paper or plastic and this moves air, generating a sound. A headphone will be capable of reproducing frequencies between 100 and 6,000 Hz, but loudspeakers can exceed this range. In order to generate lower frequencies within the audible range, more power is needed and so more air must be moved, which requires a larger cone than that of a headphone. This is the reason why most loudspeakers are 8 or more inches in diameter. But the larger cone results in a larger mass than the earphone, and this larger mass is difficult to move at high frequencies. That is, to gain low-frequency response the speaker must be large, and for high frequencies it must be small and light. To obtain both ranges, many speaker systems today have a low-frequency speaker, a *woofer,* and a high-frequency speaker, a *tweeter.* In audiometrics, however, only a single speaker is

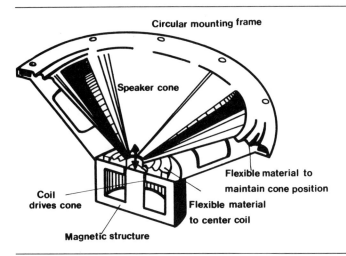

Circular mounting frame

Speaker cone

Coil drives cone

Flexible material to maintain cone position

Flexible material to center coil

Magnetic structure

FIG. 6-11.   General construction of a permanent magnet loudspeaker.

most often used because, if more than one were used, phase differences and various types of frequency distortion might arise from the filter network that routes the frequencies to the various speakers and also from the different sizes of the two speakers.

CUTTER HEADS AND VIBROTACTILE STIMULATORS

There are two output transducers that resemble the phonograph cartridge. One is the cutter head, which is the device used to cut a master recording. It is a coil of wire with a shaft and a sharp stylus connected. There are permanent magnets around the coil. When a current is fed it, the coil moves, and the sharp stylus scribes a recording pattern. (Sometimes the stylus is heated, and it then melts its way along a plastic record.)

The other device resembling the cartridge is a vibrotactile stimulator, which can be used to vibrate the skin to test tactile sensation or be used in multiple configurations to vibrate in a pattern on the skin. Figure 6-12 shows this. Braille characters can be generated, for example.

HEADPHONES
Dynamic Headphones
In general, headphones may be thought of as small loudspeakers, although their operation on the ear is somewhat different. The most common type of headphone used today is the dynamic headphone, which operates on the same principle as the dynamic loudspeaker. There is a small diaphragm to which is attached a coil. The coil is centered around a permanent magnet, and the fluctuating current in the coil causes attraction and repulsion of the coil by the magnet. This, in turn, moves the

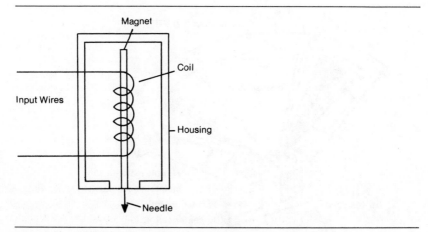

FIG. 6-12.   General construction of a vibrotactile transducer.

diaphragm and generates a sound. The major difference between loud-speakers and headphones is that the latter must be mounted on the ears, which has a great deal to do with their performance. Also, because the headphone can be coupled almost directly to the ear, the performance is often much better than with a loudspeaker.

Most modern headphones consist of a driving mechanism that is housed in a cushion. The cushion holds the driving mechanism centered approximately over the entrance to the external auditory meatus. The purpose of the driving mechanism is to create the pressure pattern of the sound represented by the electrical signal in the coil. The purposes of the cushion are (1) to hold the headphone on the head and over the ear, (2) to seal the cavity to prevent external sounds from entering, and (3) to provide a closely coupled system between earphone and tympanic membrane that, in turn, can result in excellent fidelity and high efficiency. By *closely coupled system* we mean that the diaphragm in the headphone is moving air; the pressure changes in the air are coupled directly to the tympanic membrane because the air in the canal cannot be compressed very much and so behaves as a relatively solid coupling. In a loudspeaker, the pressure changes created by the loudspeaker cone move air, but much of the pressure fluctuation in the air is dissipated before it reaches the ear. Also, in the case of the loudspeaker, the listening environment can greatly affect the performance of the loudspeaker and the fidelity with which the sound is transmitted to the ear. For example, reverberation and reflection can add additional energy peaks and troughs by causing multiple signals to add and subtract from one another. In the headphone, which is closely coupled, all of the pressure changes are coupled directly if the cushion seals the system. The result is no wasted energy.

For almost all audiometers the headphone is one designated as the TDH-49 with the MX41/AR cushion. Both of these units are derived from military designs and are heavy and somewhat uncomfortable to wear. This headphone does have the advantage of having relatively flat response within its frequency range and the ability to handle high signal levels for long periods of time. The cushion is simply a doughnut-shaped piece of rubber that presses against the pinna itself. This type of mounting does present problems for several reasons. First, not all pinnae are alike, so that the seal of the cushion often is better on one head than another. Second, there may be enough lateral variability in the system placement that the acoustic center of the driving element may not be over the external auditory meatus. In such a case, the result is that some of the sound emanating from the headphone may be directed into the wall of the canal rather than directly into the ear. Loudspeakers and headphones tend to have increased directivity at higher frequencies because of the vibrating patterns of their diaphragms. At higher frequencies a cone no longer vibrates as a whole, but in parts. As frequency is increased the sound pattern tends to be more and more focused. The result is that higher frequencies will be missing from the signal striking the tympanic membrane if the driver directs sound into the canal wall. This means that the frequency response of the headphone will not be flat. Third, as mentioned before, the headphones are heavy and uncomfortable. For listening tasks other than audiometric examinations different headphones might be used.

One new type of cushion is the circumaural cushion, which consists of a hard plastic material, in which the driving element is placed. This cushion is sufficiently large that it fits over the entire pinna and rests against the skull. The result of this is that variations in pinnae do not cause resultant changes in coupling of the headphone. Also, since the pressure of the phone is against the skull rather than against the pinna, it is more comfortable. In addition, the cushion provides more sound isolation. One particular brand of the cushion has a lining filled with plastic fluid. The fluid provides much more sound isolation than the plastic alone. (Often, these cushions are used in industrial hearing tests, where there is a great deal of environmental noise.) The cushion is also heat-sensitive so that it softens and forms to the skull through body heat. However, calibrating these cushions for audiometers has not been standardized.

There are several new designs for both headphone drivers (the transducer mechanism) and cushions that will be mentioned, since they can act as comfortable and faithful listening devices. Several systems have refined the materials in the drivers, especially the magnetic material, which has enabled designers to produce much lighter headphones capable of excellent frequency response. This has resulted in a proliferation of so-called featherweight headphones.

Crystal Headphones

Crystal headphones are uncommon, but are still used as high-impedance transducers. Also, they sometimes provide better high-frequency response than other types of output transducers. Like crystal microphones, they make use of the piezoelectric effect. In the microphone, when the cone is moved by acoustic pressure, the crystal to which it is connected is distorted and thereby generates a voltage proportional to the distortion. In the case of a crystal loudspeaker, the complement is true. In this case, when a current is applied to a crystal, the crystal is bent. One end of the crystal is attached to a solid mounting and the other end to a cone of paper. When current is applied to the crystal, it flexes and the cone is moved.

Insert Headphones

Finally the insert headphone is used in some designs. These phones consist of driving elements that are coupled to the ear by inserting a tube directly into the external auditory meatus. This eliminates all of the cushion problems, can seal the canal and eliminate external noise, and prevents much of the high-frequency loss inherent with supraaural placements. The modern high-frequency audiometer, which tests at frequencies to 18,000 kHz, makes use of these headphones. It should be mentioned here, however, that these intraaural headphones are considered very uncomfortable by most people and cause irritation of the ear after being worn for long periods.

Headphone Assessment

Because of the differences in heads and ear canals it is more difficult to evaluate headphones than loudspeakers. With a loudspeaker, the shape and size of the head and external ear (pinna) may affect the listening pattern; they do not cause a change in performance of the loudspeaker itself, just a change in the perception of the loudspeaker output. This is because both the loudspeaker and the ear are coupled to the air, but they are not directly coupled to each other. The coupling of the ear to the air being moved by a speaker influences what the ear receives but it has no influence on the speaker. The headphone, however, is directly and tightly coupled to the ear. The impedance of a headphone must be coupled to the impedance of the auditory system, and discrepant values of either will result in quite different responses. This means that a headphone may perform well on one listener because the auditory impedance is equal to the acoustic impedance of the headphone. If the same headphone is placed on another listener whose auditory impedance is different, there may be less than efficient coupling. Consequently, some compromises and variability will inevitably occur in headphone assessment.

The headphone is made to operate into the impedance of the auditory system, so it must be evaluated in that environment. To permit measurement of headphones, several techniques have been developed. One uses a device called a *flat-plate coupler.* This is essentially a flat plate of metal in the center of which is mounted a microphone element that is coupled to a sound level meter. The headphone to be assessed is placed over the microphone and various signals are fed into the headphone. The output of the headphone can then be measured with the sound level meter. This technique can certainly be used to compare one type of headphone with another, but the system bears little relationship to operation of the headphone on real ears. To provide an impedance closer to that of the auditory system, the *6-cc coupler* has been constructed. This is a metal tube enclosing 6 cc of air, which is approximately the average volume of the auditory canal in an adult. The artificial ear is designed to provide approximately the same impedance characteristics to an earphone under test as the human ear canal. This requires that the artificial ear be acoustically similar to the human ear in shape and volume and in the density characteristics of the material of its walls. How, then, can one construct an artificial ear of metal as an analog of an ear canal lined with skin? As it happens, immediately under the canal surface tissue is very dense bone. Because the tissue lining the auditory canal is so dense, the canal characteristics do not figure importantly in the impedance calculation, so that the majority of the impedance of the auditory canal is represented by the volume of air alone. That is, a coupler that mimics the volume of the ear canal and the dense tissue characteristics of the walls provides a satisfactory model. At the bottom of the tube is the microphone element as in the flat-plate coupler. It is assumed that the impedance of the microphone diaphragm is not too much different from the tympanic membrane and ossicles. There is an ANSI standard describing the construction of the 6-cc coupler to be used in measuring earphone response; in any case, the coupler provides a more valid measure of headphone performance on the human than does the flat-plate coupler.

The insert headphone is similar to the hearing-aid receiver, and the system developed for hearing-aid assessment uses a 2-cc coupler. This consists of a tube enclosing 2 cc of air, which is about the volume of the canal when an ear mold is in place. The intraaural headphone can then be coupled to this cavity and the headphone response measured as with other types of headphones. Again, there is an ANSI standard covering these couplers.

Suggested Reading

Beranek, L. L. *Acoustic Measurements.* New York: Wiley, 1962.
Crowhurst, N. H. *Basic Audio.* New York: Rider, 1959.

Everest, F. A. *Acoustic Techniques for Home and Studio.* Blue Ridge Summit, PA: TAB Books, 1984.

Geddes, L. A., and Baker, L. E. *Biomedical Instrumentation.* New York: Wiley, 1968.

Hirano, M., and Ohala, J.   Use of hooked-wire electrodes for electromyography. *J. Speech Hear. Res.* 12:362–373, 1969.

Lass, N. J. (Ed.).   *Contemporary Issues in Experimental Phonetics.* New York: Academic, 1976.

Watkins, K. L., and Zagzebski, J. A. On-line ultrasonic technique for monitoring tongue movement. *J. Acoust. Soc. Am.* 54:544–547, 1973.

7. The Meter

The meter is one of the most commonly used transducers in the laboratory. It is based on the relationship of electricity and magnetism. It converts electricity to a mechanical (rotational) movement and can be designed to measure voltage, current, or resistance.

Operating Principles

The electromagnetic principle is the basis for galvanometer movement, which is the basis of any meter. A coil of very light wire is wound around a small iron core. The core has a shaft through its axis. The shaft rests in fine jeweled pivots, as in a watch. A permanent magnet is placed around the coil, with the south pole at one side and the north at the other. Figure 7-1 illustrates this construction.

CURRENT MEASUREMENT

If a current is passed through the coil, the ends become polarized and the north end of the coil is attracted by the south pole of the magnet. Because the coil is pivoted, it is free to move under the magnetic force exerted. A pointer is attached to the moving coil and the result is a meter movement. The coil moves in direct proportion to the strength of the field set up around it by the current passing through it. Thus, the pointer moves as a function of the current flow.

In order to make the galvanometer useful it is calibrated by passing various amounts of current through the coil and noting the pointer deflection. A scale is then constructed with marks at each of the known

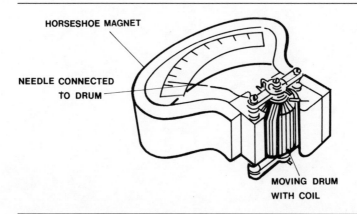

FIG. 7-1.   Basic meter construction.

points and, by interpolation, intermediate points are assigned appropriate values. The result is a meter for measuring current, called an *ammeter*. The galvanometer movement is at the heart of most meters found in the clinic and the laboratory.

To calibrate the meter it is necessary to use known values of current, but how is it possible to determine these values? The International Ampere is an amount of current that, when passed through a solution of silver nitrate, deposits 0.001118 g of silver nitrate per second. The current is determined and specified by the amount of plating deposited in a standard solution. That is, meter calibration is done by measuring the weight of silver plating in a specified period of time and converting this figure to the amount of current that must have flowed.

A meter has a limiting value of current that, when exceeded, causes no further movement of the coil. The coil has stops built into it so that the device is unable to rotate through an arc much greater than 160°. If it were allowed to move further, it could reverse itself and become stationary. Common values of limiting current are 100 μA (100 × 0.000001 A) and 1 mA. The limiting value is expressed as the current that results in the needle deflecting to its maximum point of *full scale* (FS). Most movements have the full scale value printed somewhere on the face.

Because meters are very sensitive, some additional components are necessary in order to measure large values of current. This compensation is usually done by adding *multiplier resistors*. For example, if the meter has a sensitivity of 100 μA = FS and a current of 1 A is to be measured, an extra resistor of 1-Ω value is placed in parallel with it. Figure 7-2 shows this arrangement. The meter itself will also offer some resistance to the circuit, but usually the resistance is so small we ignore it in our computations. The majority of the 1-A current passes through the 1-Ω resistor, but 100μA is allowed to flow through the meter by the 1-MΩ

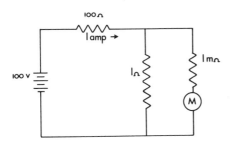

FIG. 7-2.   A circuit illustrating addition of multiplier resistors to a meter circuit.

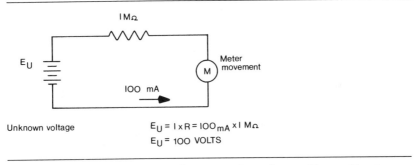

FIG. 7-3.   The circuit that exists when measuring voltage with a multimeter.

resistor. Note that the parallel combination of the 1-Ω and the 1-MΩ resistors change the total resistance of the circuit only slightly. Most ammeters are designed to measure a wide range of currents and have several multipliers, which can be selected by a switch, built in.

VOLTAGE MEASUREMENT

The galvanometer is also used to measure voltage. In this case, a resistor is placed in series with the movement. When the meter is connected to a source of EMF, a current flows, but the amount of current depends on the value of the resistor in series with the meter, as shown in Figure 7-3. For example, with the 100 μA = FS movement and a resistor of 1 MΩ, 100 μA flows through the meter when connected to 100 V. Therefore, the face of the meter could be labeled as measuring voltage rather than current, and the full scale value would be 100 V. Again, as in the case of the ammeter, several multipliers are switch-selectable so that a wide range of voltages can be measured.

RESISTANCE MEASURMENT

To adapt the galvanometer for measuring resistance, a source of voltage is built into the meter along with multipliers. Usually the voltage source is a dry cell of 1.5 V. If this arrangement is connected to a resistor of 15 kilohms, 100 μA flows. The meter could then be calibrated and the full scale point would be labeled as 15 kilohms. In order to measure smaller resistances, additional multipliers are added so that at no time can the meter receive more than 100 μA of current.

MULTIMETERS

A *multimeter* is a device that contains a movement and all the necessary multipliers and a source of voltage for measuring current, voltage, or resistance.

A caution in using meters for measuring current: if a meter is placed into a circuit carrying significantly more current than the meter can take, the current may burn out the meter movement by heating and burning out the coil wire or may ruin the meter by causing the pointer to bang against its maximum stop so hard that the pointer bends or snaps off. Therefore, current is always measured by setting the meter range–switch to the largest value of current and stepping down through the ranges until the appropriate range is found.

To repeat, the same meter can be calibrated to measure voltage rather than current because the current in a branch of a circuit is a single value, but the voltage drop (E) across any component in that branch is determined by the current flowing (I) and the resistance (R) of the component ($E = I/R$). To measure voltage, the meter must parallel the component(s) across which the voltage drop will be measured. That is, the meter actually becomes a branch paralleling the component(s) it will measure.

Changing the amount of resistance in the meter branch (i.e., the size of a precision resistor in series with the meter movement) changes the proportion of current that will flow in the meter as a branch paralleling the circuit being measured, and so alters the range of voltages being measured.

And finally, the same meter can be used to measure resistance of an element. In this case, the element must be removed from a circuit since it becomes part of a circuit involving the meter itself and a voltage supply. If the element whose resistance is to be measured is not removed from its circuit, the measurement may actually include other branches of the circuit. The resistance to be measured is placed into a circuit of a voltage source (typically a battery), plus the meter, plus the unknown. The battery supplies some voltage (e.g., 1.5 V, 6 V, or 9 V), and the current drawn by the circuit is determined by the total resistance of the circuit, that is, the resistance of the meter plus the unknown resistance. If the meter is designed to read full-scale for some specified current (and, therefore, some specified resistance), the meter dial can be calibrated to read the contribution that arises from the unknown. As discussed previously, different ranges of resistances can be measured so that in each case a known magnitude of meter movement arises from the total circuit resistance, but the meter is labeled by that part contributed by the unknown resistance.

Other Meters

ALTERNATING CURRENT

Thus far we have been discussing the measurement of direct current (DC) quantities, but in speech and hearing we are most often measuring varying quantities: alternating current (AC) within the audio range. Obviously we cannot connect a galvanometer movement directly to an AC circuit because the meter would be driven first in one direction and then in the other as a function of the direction of current flow through the meter coil. What usually happens is that the meter does not appear to move at all: the change in current direction is too rapid for the meter to begin to follow. Some signal processing must be done so that the meter will be able to measure the signal.

One of the simplest techniques used in meters for measuring AC is to change the current from AC to DC. A diode is a device that allows current to flow in only one direction. If an AC were fed to a diode, the output might appear as in Figure 7-4. If two or more diodes are connected in certain configurations with a transformer, the output would appear as in Figure 7-5. If this varying output is connected to a resistor-capacitor (RC) network, and if the time constant of the RC network is properly chosen, the output will be smoothed out and will approach an ideal DC without any ripple in the peaks. This value, then, can be readily measured with a galvanometer movement. The previous circuit is commonly used in meters for measuring AC voltage. (Current in AC circuits is difficult to measure, especially because the meter must be connected in series and any change in the signal will be reflected in the circuit as a whole, which is an undesirable condition.)

There is one major problem in the AC voltmeter just discussed. In order to eliminate the ripple, an RC network is used. Note that we said

FIG. 7-4.   AC voltage (E) input and output of a half-wave rectifier or diode.

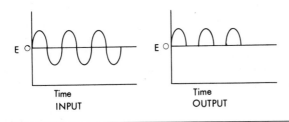

| Time | Time |
| INPUT | OUTPUT |

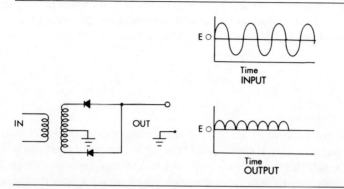

FIG. 7-5.   Full-wave circuit and associated AC voltage (E) input and output.

that the time constant of this RC network had to be *properly chosen.* But with an AC, the time constant will have different effects with different frequencies (Fig. 7-6). With low frequencies, the capacitor has sufficient time to charge and the value across it is very nearly the full value of the peak of the AC. But with higher frequencies, the capacitor never gets a chance to charge to the full AC value. This means that if the signal is rapidly changing, the value indicated on the meter will be less than if the signal is a low frequency. We now discover that the meter just discussed will often give erroneous readings for varying frequencies.

VOLUME UNIT METERS

The most common application of the AC meter is in controlling the input to various devices. The best example of this is the control of recording level to a tape recorder. If the signal input exceeds a specific voltage, the machine will distort this signal. For this reason, a volume unit (VU) meter is commonly inserted in tape-recorder circuitry, usually in the record amplifier. The specifications of the VU meter are quite rigid and are published in an IRE document (53 IRE 3.52). In theory, all meters labeled VU will respond to a specific signal in the same manner. The designers have specified the electrical characteristics of the meter, know in advance what the error will be for various speech signals, and design accordingly. So long as we all operate with the same inaccuracy we are essentially calibrated.

The specifications of any VU meter include the particulars of how it is incorporated into a circuit, the impedance across which it is to be connected, and the range of signals that may be fed to it. Also, the specifications include details concerning the impedance of the movement, the ballistics of the movement (how the needle moves in response to various waves), and the electrical characteristics of the diodes built into the meter. The reader should also be aware of the fact that many meters labeled VU are not, in fact, VU meters. A VU meter is an expensive device, and it

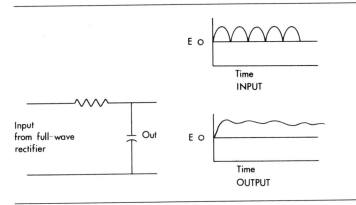

FIG. 7-6.   Ripple filter circuit and associated voltage (E) input and output.

is often easy for a designer to save money by specifying cheap movements without the proper specifications but with labels printed in volume units.

By using more sophisticated electronic processing, more modern general-purpose meters have eliminated some of the problems mentioned
previously. The variation in meter indication due to varying frequency
can be compensated for with equalizing filters. Although we have not
mentioned it previously, insensitivity of the meter movement itself is
often a handicap, so amplifiers are added before the meter movement.
Because these amplifiers are constructed using vacuum tubes, the instrument as a whole is labeled as a vacuum tube voltmeter (VTVM).

VTVMs sometimes read the value equivalent to the peak of the AC
wave. There are several problems inherent in this type of meter when
monitoring other than continuous AC waves. Speech, for example, is a
rapidly changing series of pulse-like signals. The peak values of speech
waves bear little correlation to the actual amount of energy flow. The
rate of flow of energy is the important value when discussing such waves,
so the root-mean-square meter has been developed.

ROOT-MEAN-SQUARE METERS

The root-mean-square (RMS) value of a wave is essentially the mean
value of the area between the envelope of a wave and the zero axis. For
example, the RMS value of the sine wave shown in Figure 7-7 would be
equal to the average value of the crosshatched area of the wave without
regard to sign. It should be obvious that this is a more accurate indication
of the work that could be performed than is the peak value, as the peak
only occurs for an instant twice each cycle (once + and once −).

Because the RMS value of a sine wave is equal to 0.707 times the peak
value, early RMS meters were simply peak-responding meters with the
markings on the dial changed to 0.707 of their original value: the sine-

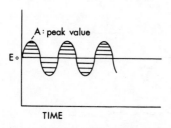

FIG. 7-7.   Total value of voltage shown as crosshatched area (RMS = 0.707 × the peak amplitude [A]).

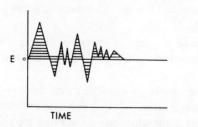

FIG. 7-8.   An aperiodic wave and its total voltage (E) shown crosshatched.

wave RMS/value. But with any wave other than a sine wave, there can be a great deal of error. Consider a speech wave as shown in Figure 7-8. The peak is very narrow and seldom occurs, so there would probably be a great deal of error in measuring this. Later versions of the RMS meter have been called *true RMS voltmeters* and do, in fact, measure the accurate RMS value by literally performing the integration and taking the mean of the integrated value.

Common Problems With Meters

Some people have said that meter-reading is an art because it is necessary to interpolate between the markings to arrive at a correct value. Also, parallax can result in error. Parallax comes about when a meter is viewed from an angle. The needle rests slightly above the surface of the meter face, so that if the device is viewed from the side, slight misreading can occur.

In some meters, a mirror is provided along part of the arc of the meter dial. When viewing such a mirrored meter, the operator places himself in such a position that he cannot see a reflection of the needle. This means that the line of sight is directly perpendicular to the meter; thus, no parallax!

Finally, one of the biggest problems with galvanometer movements is the ballistics of the meter. If the meter is to respond to rapid changes in signal, the needle should have very little mass. However, the masses of the coil and needle often limit the response quite a bit. This is especially true of speech signals because they are impulsive signals. That is, there are sudden bursts of energy, as in plosives, followed by steady-state signals such as vowels. If a meter is to respond with reasonable fidelity to the transient signals, it must have very low mass.

Several techniques have been used to obtain a meter movement with less mass that is capable of responding to rapidly changing signals. One of the earliest attempts made use of a very light metal mirror glued to the meter shaft. In this device, called a *mirror galvanometer*, a beam of light is directed at the mirror and its reflection is aimed at a scale on the wall. Because the beam is directed at a distant surface there is an amplification of the deflection of the mirror that results in an increase in sensitivity of the meter. That is, because of the distance the beam of light travels from the mirror to the meter face, a lever action results in a greater movement of the spot of light than that provided by the meter coil itself.

Electronic Meters

As yet another alternative, engineers have sought a mass-free indicating system. One of these systems has been the *neon lamp*. A neon lamp is a device containing two electrodes immersed in neon gas. If the voltage difference between the two electrodes is sufficient, the neon gas will begin to conduct current and will therefore glow.

The usual application of this indicating device is in tape recording in which the signal fed to the tape must be above a certain minimum level but not exceed a somewhat higher maximum level. In this case, the neon lamp circuit is adjusted so that the level fed to one lamp is always above the minimum input necessary for adequate recording (the lamp is always on). The next lamp is set so that the level never exceeds the minimum (the lamp does not glow) when operating properly, but the voltage between the electrodes is sufficient to cause ionization when the signal fed to the tape exceeds the safe minimum. The result is a lamp that will glow only when the level is too high. The operator then need only set the controls on the tape machine so that the second lamp almost, but not quite, glows. Such a system is essentially inertia-free and is commonly found on older tape machines.

This general idea has led to the development of an entirely new system

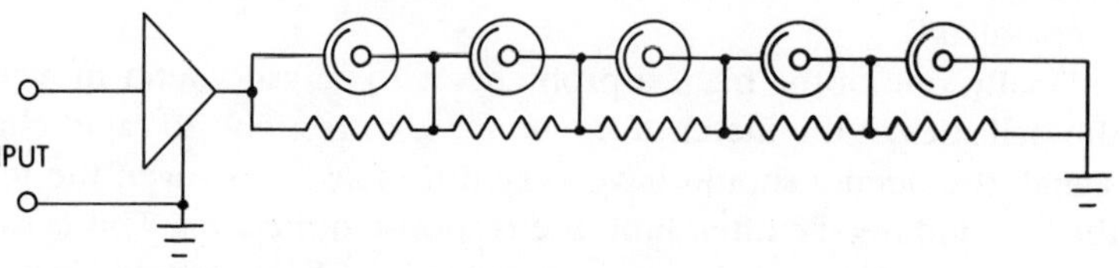

FIG. 7-9.   Level indicator using neon lamps.

of meters consisting of strings of neon tubes whose ionizing thresholds are spaced a specific number of units (often decibels) apart. A general schematic is shown in Figure 7-9. The input level at which each neon tube ionizes is increased, proceeding from left to right, so that those to the left fire at lower levels and those to the right at progressively higher levels. The result is a line of lights that varies in length as the input signal varies. The line is longest for the most intense signals. In this case it is possible to read the peak level of a signal with a great deal of precision, provided the lights stay on long enough. (Some off-time delay is built into the system so that even though the input peak may be of very short duration the lamp comes on almost immediately but has a slight lag in going off. This lag provides the user with enough time to recognize that the light is on.)

A further development in measuring instruments is the *digital voltmeter*. Since the digital voltmeter is found in many labs we will introduce this general topic by describing one in particular. Figure 7-10 is an example. Notice that the face contains a row of knobs and also a line of numbers. The numbers represent the voltage of the input signal. This type of display eliminates the problems of parallax, interpolation, and inertia because the reading is done electronically. Most of the inexpensive versions of this instrument make use of an integrated circuit generating a frequency proportional to the input voltage. That is, the integrated circuit is a voltage-to-frequency converter. This circuit chip is then combined with a frequency counter and a chip that turns on various line segments making up numerals.

Figure 7-11 is a schematic of the system. The input signal causes the V-to-F converter to operate, generating a frequency. The output of the chip is then counted for a constant duration determined by the timer. The interval is not critical so long as it remains constant and is long enough to eliminate errors due to sampling. The counter then feeds the driver chip with a number that is decoded and by illuminating various segments, provides numerals on the face of the instrument. The device can be devised to display a + or −, dependent on the input signal, and also can measure the voltage without changing any range switch. So long

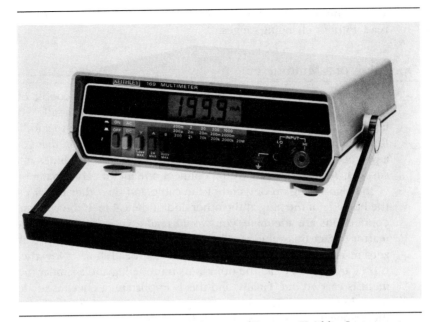

FIG. 7-10.   A high-quality digital multimeter. (Courtesy Keithley Instruments, Inc.)

FIG. 7-11.   Block diagram of one system used in digital voltmeters.

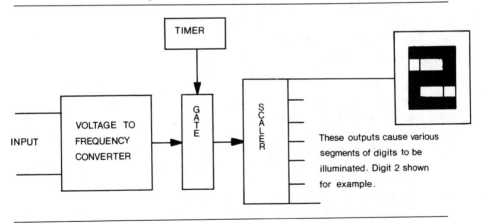

as the input is within the range of the V-to-F converter, the meter can be read without changing ranges.

Operation of a Multimeter

To clarify the operation of a multimeter let us look at a couple of situations that might be encountered in the laboratory. For example, you may be attempting to dub a tape-recording from one machine to another and find that nothing seems to be happening. If you are certain that you have a prerecorded tape, then the cable between the two machines might be suspect. To test this, you would connect one meter cable to the hot side of the signal plug on one end of the cable and the other meter cable to the hot side of the plug at the other end of the cable. If the wire and plug connections are adequate, you would read a very small resistance. As a matter of fact this value may be so small that it may appear that there is zero resistance. This is called, in the trade, a "dead short." Now the meter cables are moved to all the other pins on the plug and a similar measurement is carried out. Finally, and this is important, a check is made to all the other pins while one meter cable is connected to the hot side. If there appears to be a short circuit between the hot pin and other pins it could be that the signal is being shorted out rather than not being carried through the cable. It is sometimes a good idea to flex the cable while making these checks of continuity, since sometimes there is a break in the cable only when the cable is in a certain position.

Another use of the multimeter is to check for power in the laboratory. For example, you may be trying to operate a machine and find that the power light does not go on. You are certain the machine is plugged into the wall socket and that the switch is in the on position. What now? It may be that a fuse is blown in the laboratory wiring. To test this, you could insert the meter cable ends into the socket in the wall. This should be done very carefully and might be avoided by simply connecting one cable to the wall plate, if the latter is metal, and inserting the other cable into the socket. The meter should be set on AC volts with a range of at least 125 V. The meter should indicate an AC voltage when the cable is in one part of the socket because the house power is connected to a hot wire and a ground, which is the metal wall plate to which you have connected the meter. The other pin on the wall socket is also ground, so you should not read any voltage when the meter is connected to that since you are connecting both meter cables to ground.

Suggested Reading

Beranek, L. L. *Acoustic Measurements.* New York: Wiley, 1962.
VanValkenburgh, Nooger, and Neville, Inc. *Basic Electronics.* New York: Rider, 1955.

8. Display Devices

A variety of devices are used in the laboratory and clinic to display signals or measures taken on signals, but they may be classified into two general types: permanent displays (called hard-copy) and transient displays.

Permanent Displays

STRIP-CHART RECORDERS

A strip-chart recorder is a combination of a galvanometer movement with a pen point, instead of a needle indicator, and a paper drive. The meter movement is coupled to the pen point to move the pen across the paper as the meter movement rotates under the influence of a varying electromagnetic field. The paper drive moves a roll of paper under the pen point at some constant rate. If the pen point is not moving, because the meter is not energized or is energized to some constant value, the pen draws a straight line on the paper parallel with the paper's edge. If the constant value is altered to a different constant value, the pen will move across the paper to a new lateral location and draw out a straight line at this new location. If the variable being measured shows continuing variation, the pen will draw out a record of the variations as the point moves back and forth across the paper. If the paper is not moving, the variation will appear only as a single arc line that is created by the pen moving back and forth with the signal variation.

Because of the geometry of the system, early strip-chart recordings yielded arcs on the paper as the pen moved. Considering that a galvanometer is a rotating device, the reason that arcs were drawn is obvious.

These recordings of arcs are sometimes difficult to read, and a rectilinear record seems to be easier to interpret, if only because most graphs are rectilinear. Consequently, machines made in the last 15 years have additional mechanical linkage between the galvanometer and the pen so that the recording is rectilinear.

The strip-chart recorder has a limited frequency response that is unlikely to exceed 50 or 100 Hz. This severe limitation in its use is a result of its mechanical construction. The meter movement must be sturdy enough to support a pen and ink supply at its tip, but this mass at the end of the meter arm cannot be altered in direction fast enough to respond to higher frequencies. (*Inertia* is the name given to the reaction of a mass to variations in the force propelling it. Mass, in the mechanical domain, responds analogously to inductance in the electrical domain— inductance offers progressively more opposition to progressively higher frequencies.) That is, today higher frequencies require faster and faster changes in direction, and the more massive a body is, the harder it is for it to change direction rapidly. The larger the mass, the more energy is used in altering its direction or its velocity rapidly. (Think about trying to turn a sharp corner on a bicycle or changing lanes in a car at high speed.)

Frequently, the motor driving the paper is mechanically coupled to an oscillator (a generator of signals varying in frequency), providing an input signal to the equipment under test so that the signal frequency delivered to the test equipment varies systematically. (Most likely, the particular type of strip-chart recorder used in equipment evaluation is the graphic level recorder, discussed below, because of its special characteristics, but the principles hold for any strip-chart recorder.) If the chart paper is calibrated to note the signal frequency, one can test the frequency response of a system by graphing the output of the system continuously while sweeping through any frequency band of interest. Fig. 8-1 shows this arrangement (the dotted line in the figure indicates that the signal generator dial and the chart paper are driven together). Fig. 8-2 is a frequency-response plot of a microphone and is an example of a plot of the output of a microphone as the frequency of the signal into the microphone is varied from low to high.

The mirror galvanometer principle, discussed in Chapter 7, has also been used in chart recording devices. One such instrument makes use of light-sensitive paper moved past the mirror, which is connected to the meter movement instead of a pen. When the light beam is aimed at the paper, it exposes the film and the deflection of the mirror is recorded on the paper. Devices making use of the light beam indicator can record signals up to about 200 Hz, which is a great improvement over pen recorders but still is not adequate to record higher frequency audio signals.

To improve further the frequency-response capabilities of chart recorders, engineers have made use of the cathode-ray tube, which will be

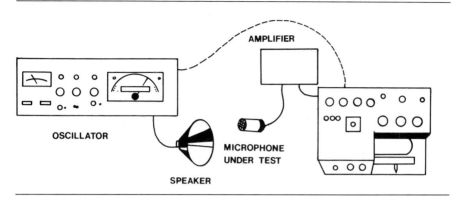

FIG. 8-1. Equipment arrangement for measuring frequency response of an amplifier. The dotted line is a flexible shaft connecting the oscillator and the response plotter together so that as frequency from the oscillator changes, the graph paper moves to a different position.

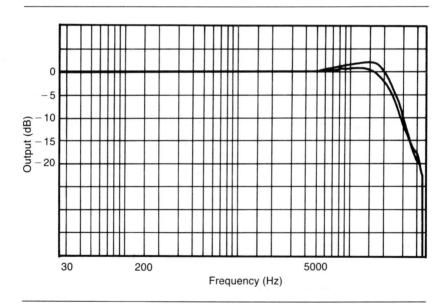

FIG. 8-2. Typical frequency response chart of a high-quality microphone.

described later, fiber optics (fiber optics are light conductors), and strip charts of photographic paper. It should be obvious, however, that a strip-chart recorder can be used only for relatively slow events and where low frequency information is desired. The special strip chart that records in decibels—the graphic level recorder—finds use in the evaluation of equipment such as hearing aid systems and in special applications such as industrial noise surveys.

GRAPHIC LEVEL RECORDERS

One particular type of strip-chart recorder serves quite a different purpose from most others. The graphic level recorder differs because it incorporates an amplifier that is insensitive to momentary variations in waveform. Instead, it represents the average amplitude (over some small time constant) of a signal but not its waveform. Furthermore, the amplifier causes the pen to deflect as a logarithmic function of amplitude of the signal, and the graphic record represents amplitude in decibels. One further difference in some graphic level recorders is that the pen is not controlled by a galvanometer but operates through an amplifier with feedback; this difference is complicated and of little general interest here.

X-Y RECORDERS

The X-Y recorder is unlike a strip-chart recorder in that it uses a stationary piece of paper. The pen point can be moved to any location on the surface by a combination of voltages delivered to a horizontal deflection amplifier (on the X axis) and a vertical deflection amplifier (on the Y axis). A permanent ink record is made of the pen movement as it displays the simultaneous variations in the signal fed to the two amplifiers as in, for example, the X-Y recorders used in tympanometry.

The X-Y plotter is used with any system that requires an X-Y output, such as tympanometry or evoked response audiometry. Many computer applications also lend themselves to effective X-Y displays.

Transient Displays

OSCILLOSCOPES

The oscilloscope is a device that can display waveforms instantaneously and, in some cases, even store them for a long period of time. Until about 40 years ago, the only method available for displaying waveforms was the strip-chart recorder. This technique provides a permanent record, but, as noted earlier, higher frequency response is severely limited because of inertial lag due to the masses of the pen and of the parts of the galvanometer movement. The oscilloscope eliminates this problem because the moving element providing the picture is a beam of electrons, which is essentially massless.

Not only is the oscilloscope essentially free of frequency limitations for audio frequencies, but a good laboratory oscilloscope offers a very wide variety of uses: voltage measurements can be taken, signals can be timed or compared with one another, signal purity can be examined, or the linearity (freedom from distortion) of a total system or any component can be appraised. Because of all these and other potential uses, the oscilloscope is of almost ubiquitous assistance in the laboratory and thus will be considered here in enough detail to give the reader an appreciation of its operation, its components, and the options it allows.

Operating Principles

The principal element in the oscilloscope is the *cathode-ray tube* (CRT). The CRT consists of a large vacuum tube with a heated cathode at one end. Electrons are boiled off the hot cathode and attracted to the other end of the tube by a very high positive voltage there. (This voltage may be from 10,000 to 75,000 V, so the clinician is urged to stay out of the case of an oscilloscope. Maintenance of this instrument is best left to an electronics technician.) The inside face of the CRT is coated with a phosphor which emits a spot of light each time that it is struck by a moving electron. Thus, if a beam of electrons moves across the screen (the back of the faceplate) a line will result. Fig. 8-3 is a side view of the CRT. The focusing coil is a device that concentrates the beam of electrons from the cathode ray gun and prevents them from spreading on the way to the faceplate, resulting in a sharp dot rather than a fuzzy one. The deflection plates consist of two sets of elements, one set above and below the beam and another to either side of it. The plates above and below, called the *vertical deflection plates,* can have either positive or negative values on

FIG. 8-3.   Schematic construction of cathode-ray tube (CRT). VDP = vertical deflection plate; HDP = horizontal deflection plate.

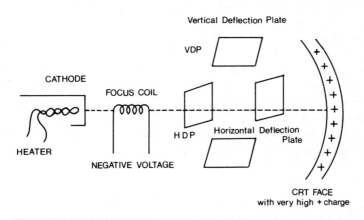

them. If they have neither, the beam will move straight from the cathode in the center of the screen. If the plate above has a positive value on it, the beam will be attracted to it on the way to the CRT face. If the plate below has a negative voltage on it, the beam will be repelled in the same direction, as if the top plate were pulling it. Thus, the beam can be moved up or down depending on the voltage applied. Any signal applied to the vertical amplifier, which in turn is connected to the vertical deflection plates, will then be displayed as an up or down deflection of the beam.

The same is true of the other two plates, called the *horizontal deflection plates.* The horizontal plates, which create horizontal movement of the beam, are significant contributors to the utility of the CRT because, in its typical use, the beam travels across the face of the oscilloscope in a precisely calibrated amount of time, allowing for a variety of time and frequency measurements of the signals displayed on the screen. Therefore, the oscilloscope becomes useful for examining and calibrating signals.

To obtain precise calibration of the beam travel, the oscilloscope must deliver some voltage to the horizontal plates. This voltage pulls the beam all the way to the left (as viewed from the front) and then evenly and smoothly pulls the beam to the right in some fixed amount of time. When the beam has traveled all the way to the right, it must be returned to the left instantaneously and then pulled right again at the calibrated rate.

Pulling the beam to the right smoothly requires a constantly increasing positive voltage to the right horizontal deflection plate and a constantly decreasing positive or increasing negative voltage to the left horizontal deflection plate. Fig. 8-4 shows a sawtooth wave that might be applied to a deflection plate. As the voltage becomes positive, the electron beam is attracted—the attraction increasing as the voltage becomes increasingly positive. At the peak voltage, the beam is attracted maximally and is deflected all the way to the right. Then the voltage suddenly becomes very negative, the beam snaps back to the left because it is being repelled, and the cycle is repeated.* Returning the base to the left edge requires returning the voltages from their values with the beam full right to their values with the beam full left but doing so instantaneously. When this repeated control voltage is itself displayed, as in Fig. 8-4, the result is the sawtooth wave. If the period of the sawtooth wave is precisely calibrated, then one can measure temporal aspects of any displayed signal. For this reason, the horizontal plate controls are typically labeled the *time base* and frequently give the user a switch with a series of ranges of time windows. The vertical plates are amplitude-controlled by the signal being investigated, so the result is a waveform. That is, the beam is

---

*Simultaneously with the return of the beam an internal signal is generated that shuts off the beam during its return trip. This prevents a beam travelling from right to left, which would only clutter the oscilloscope.

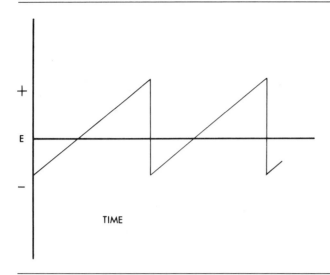

FIG. 8-4.   Sawtooth waveform as used for the time base in an oscilloscope. E = voltage.

deflected up and down by the input voltage just as the beam is deflected right to left by the internal sawtooth.

Fig. 8-5 shows the front of a typical oscilloscope. There are three sets of controls: the *beam adjustments,* the *vertical amplifier,* and the *time base* (horizontal amplifier).

The beam adjustments consist of variable resistors that control the brightness of the spot of light, the focus of the spot, and a control that determines the roundness of the spot. The latter is called the *astigmatism control,* but not all oscilloscopes have this control. It is best to keep the brightness at a minimum when not using the oscilloscope, and it is absolutely necessary to keep it turned off when the beam is not moving; otherwise, the beam may strike one spot for too long a period of time and burn a spot permanently on the face. Most users energize the time base when no signal is being delivered to the oscilloscope, so that a line appears across the screen as the beam sweeps repeatedly across the face.

The vertical amplifier receives the external signal and amplifies it sufficiently to drive the vertical deflection plates. Note that the controls are calibrated so that for a given amount of deflection, measured in centimeters, the voltage input can be determined. The better the oscilloscope quality, the better will be that calibration, so that scopes easily serve as meters for measuring voltage and its analogs precisely.

The horizontal beam is controlled by a time base that is a sawtooth wave generator and an amplifier. The rate of the generator determines the speed with which the beam is pulled across the screen. Some oscil-

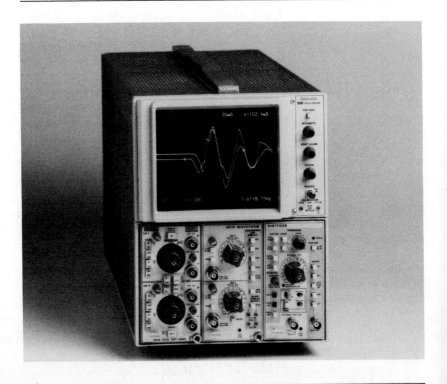

FIG. 8-5.   A two-channel digital oscilloscope. (Courtesy Tektronix, Inc.)

loscopes have provisions for feeding an external signal to the vertical plates. This signal is sometimes used to generate Lissajous patterns, which give an indication of the similarity between two waves. The Lissajous pattern is truly a continuous correlation coefficient. If the waves fed to both the horizontal and vertical plates are identical in frequency, amplitude, and phase, the pattern will be a diagonal line across the scope, with a slope of 45°. If they differ in amplitude, the slope will be different from 45°. If the signals differ in phase, the pattern will be elliptical or circular or, if the waves are exactly 180° out of phase, a straight line, but one with an opposite slope from the identical wave situation. If the signals differ in frequency, the pattern will change, depending on the frequency difference.

The oscilloscope is used by simply connecting the external signal to the vertical amplifier, selecting an appropriate sweep rate (the rate at which the internal sawtooth wave is generated), turning the unit on, and adjusting the various beam controls for the best-looking pattern. The knobs associated with the sweep generator or time base are calibrated in millimeters per second or centimeters per second, and the vertical amplifier is calibrated in volts per centimeter. By noting the setting of the controls and measuring the number of millimeters the beam is deflected, the period of a wave or the voltage of a wave may be determined. It is a simple matter to determine the frequency (f) of a wave once the period (p) is determined because the relationship f = 1/p holds true. The vertical amplifier can be used to determine the sensitivity of the input transducer so that the relationship between the measured voltage and the input pressure, flow, or displacement can be calculated.

There is another set of controls, called the *trigger controls*, that may be necessary at times. These allow the trace via the sweep generator to be triggered by a choice of signals: the signal to be displayed, the 60-Hz line voltage, or an external pulse. When the trigger circuit is being used, there is no trace on the screen until the trigger is activated. This arrangement is useful in, for example, looking at the rapid onset of a tone. The trigger is used so that the sweep begins just as the tone begins and allows the operator to look at the beginning of the waveform. In the case of repetitive signals, the trigger will seem to freeze the image if the visualized wave starts at the same point on the input wave each time.

Some very expensive oscilloscopes have a storage function that allows a waveform to be held on the screen for hours or even days. This is made possible by using a special CRT and its accompanying controls. These controls are shown in Fig. 8-6. The *store* button activates the storage feature so that the CRT no longer functions as a normal CRT, but can now store signals. Usually the trigger function is used with the *single sweep function,* which provides for a single sweep to go into storage. The storage feature allows that one sweep to be viewed repeatedly. Only a single sweep is stored at one time; otherwise, the feature of interest might be obscured by a buildup of many sweeps.

The reader should understand that the storage oscilloscope is not the same as a signal averaging device, which includes an oscilloscope. The storage oscilloscope displays any signal fed into it so that if repeated signals are delivered, it will display all of them. Should signals differ markedly from one another, the screen of the oscilloscope will likely show a white blur as the increasing number of signals are repeatedly displayed. A *signal averager,* on the other hand, is a storage device incorporating an oscilloscope in its output. For repeated signal delivery, the averager sums the waveforms and displays a single waveform output on the oscilloscope's face; this waveform is the algebraic sum of all the previous inputs. This means that any random signals will usually sum to zero because each positive signal will probably be cancelled by an equivalent negative signal over a long period of time, whereas a constant, recurring positive signal will be enhanced over time. This designation of these machines as *averagers* is perhaps a mistake.

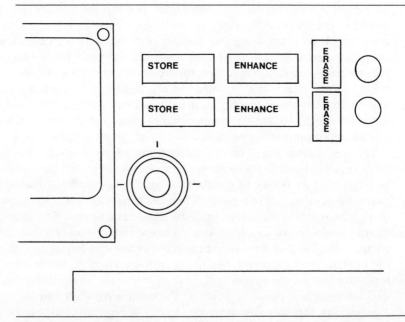

FIG. 8-6.   The storage and erase controls on an oscilloscope. The screen is to the left of the store buttons.

The *enhance* button essentially controls the contrast on the screen and is used at high sweep rates. The *erase* button erases waveform patterns from the screen.

There are so many different types of oscilloscopes available today for such a wide variety of uses that a comprehensive discussion of them all is beyond the range of this book. For this reason, the user should try a variety of applications of the oscilloscope, following the instructions in the manual provided by the manufacturer.

Special Features
All the characteristics that have been discussed to this point are universal to oscilloscopes. Most oscilloscopes also offer a variety—typically a wide variety—of additional capacities that contribute heavily to the general utility of oscilloscopes in any laboratory.

The basic use of the oscilloscope in visually portraying the waveshape of any signal that varies over time is realized by feeding the signal to the vertical plates, during which the horizontal plates are fed a carefully controlled sawtooth waveform. This results in the signal moving across the face of the oscilloscope's screen at some constant rate. If the repetition rate of the sawtooth wave is 100 per second, for example, then each one-hundredth of the second will be portrayed as a separate sweep. These sweeps will be superimposed on one another so that one or more will appear simultaneously. (Whether there will be simultaneous appearance is determined by the characteristics of the coating on the screen of the cathode-ray tube—some coatings result in a slow fading phosphorescence while others fade more rapidly. Often a laboratory will own more than one cathode-ray tube for an oscilloscope, allowing a choice among tubes having longer or shorter visualization times.)

If the signal being portrayed is repetitive, and if the sweep time of the scope (the repetition rate of the sawtooth wave controlling the sweep) is continuously variable, then one or more cycles of the signal on the face of the oscilloscope can be frozen by adjusting the sweep time so that each new sweep begins at the same point on the signal as the last sweep and exactly the same waveform is repeatedly displayed.

More or fewer cycles of the signal can be displayed by decreasing or increasing the sawtooth (timing cycle of the sweep) wave repetition rate. The fewer cycles displayed on the scope, the greater the detail that can be seen in the signal waveform. Because of this, a major use of the oscilloscope is in examining waveforms in detail.

Typically, the oscilloscope will have a grid overlaid on the face, which is carefully etched and frequently edge-lighted with an adjustable magnitude of illumination. The detail of the wave can be examined against the markings of the grid, which is called a *reticule* and resembles graph paper.

If the amplitude of a signal displayed between the vertical plates is carefully calibrated and controlled and is accurately displayed at the control knob, another use of the scope is as a voltage meter.

Often it is desirable to examine two tonal sources to ensure that they are identical in frequency or to set them to be identical and to determine or set their phase relation. This can be done easily in either of two ways, one of which is to put one signal on the horizontal plates and the other on the vertical plates. The resulting display is the Lissajous figure that for two identical frequencies bears a particular form determined by the phase relationship of the inputs. The alternative way is to display both signals between the vertical plates. With some oscilloscopes, it is possible to display both signals because the scope is built with two separate beams so that one signal is displayed on each. This type of oscilloscope is called a *dual-beam oscilloscope*. With most oscilloscopes that are not dual-beam, the scope circuitry allows display of two signals because it includes a circuit that rapidly and alternately samples each signal, displaying one signal above the other. Each signal is actually presented as a dashed line, but the alternation rate is sufficiently high that the eye sees each signal as a separate fused image. The dual-beam oscilloscope allows control of the vertical location of each signal on the CRT so that the two can be displayed (one over the other or superimposed on the other, for example) for examination and contrast. The ability of a dual-beam oscil-

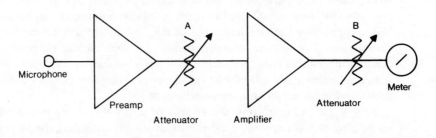

FIG. 8-7.   Block diagram of a sound level meter.

loscope to display two signals simultaneously makes it an appropriate device for visual examination of both the input and the output of a piece of equipment (e.g., a hearing aid), tracing of a signal through a piece of equipment, and so forth.

Oscilloscopes also often allow the display of transient events by providing what is called an external trigger. The trigger circuit holds the beam just off the face of the oscilloscope to the left. The signal line is fed into the trigger input and the signal itself serves as the release of the beam, which then moves from left to right, displaying the transient event itself as it lights the screen.

SOUND LEVEL METERS

The sound level meter (SLM) is becoming a very useful instrument for the speech pathologist as well as for the audiologist. The SLM provides a simple estimate of the intensity of a speaking voice and thus has proved useful in voice therapy. With the background the reader has already acquired from this book, he or she should be able to determine the construction of the instrument in general, if not in detail.

To measure the intensity of a sound, the acoustic signal must be transduced to an electrical signal by means of a microphone. The weak signal from the microphone is amplified and the resulting electrical signal is connected to a voltmeter that is calibrated in terms of decibels giving the sound pressure level. In order to extend the range of the meter so that both extremely weak and extremely intense signals can be read, an attenuator is included in the circuit. As a matter of fact, many SLMs use two attenuators, one between the preamplifier and the amplifier and one just before the meter. The reason for this, as discussed in Chapter 3, is that the signal-to-noise ratio can be degraded if the attenuator is placed too early in the circuit, so that the ideal place is just prior to the output; thus, one attenuator is placed at this position. However, if the SLM is to measure signals between about 30 dB and 130 dB the amplifier must have a great deal of gain for the weak signals, but strong signals can overload an amplifier with such sensitivity. Therefore, an additional attenua-

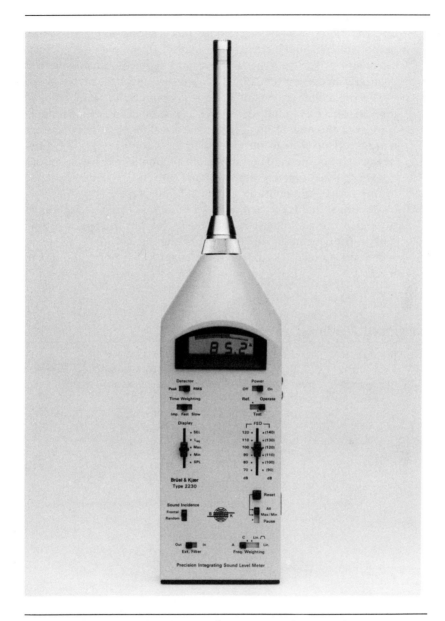

FIG. 8-8.   Modern sound level meter. (Courtesy Bruel & Kjaer Instruments, Inc., Marlborough, Mass.)

tor is placed just before the amplifier so that intense signals cannot over-load the meter. A block diagram for this is shown in Fig. 8-7. For signals of moderate to high intensity, the input to the amplifier is attenuated by attenuator A. For weak signals in which the maximum amount of ampli-fication is needed, attenuator B is used to control the meter input.

The preceding attenuator pattern is common in many amplifier sys-tems that have extreme amounts of gain (about 100 dB or more).

Most of the new SLMs operate without the necessity of setting atten-uators, relying instead on electronic gain control. Fig. 8-8 shows one newer type of meter. The output of the amplifier drives a set of digital converters that convert the AC signal into binary coded decimals that, in turn, drive light-emitting diode (LED) displays.

Modern sound level meters provide quite a variety of additional func-tions that the audiologist might find useful, but the speech pathologist will probably be interested only in reading the instantaneous sound pres-sure level. Consult any of the many manufacturers for additional infor-mation.

Suggested Readings

Beranek, L. L.   *Acoustic Measurements.* New York: Wiley, 1962.

Crowhurst, N. H.   *Audio Measurements.* New York: Gernsback, 1958.

Flanagan, J. L.   *Speech Analysis, Synthesis, and Perception.* New York: Springer-Verlag, 1965.

9. Tape Recorders and Recording

Operating Principles of Tape Recording

If a tape that has a metal oxide deposit on it is moved past a coil in which an alternating current (AC) is flowing, the oxide particles on the tape will become magnetized. When this magnetized tape is passed by another coil that is passive, a current will be induced in the coil. If this induced current is passed through a resistor and the resultant electromotive force (EMF) is amplified, the same pattern of electron motion is created as existed in the original coil. This is the basic operating principle of the modern tape recorder. All the differences among available machines, then, are in coil design, characteristic tape format, and control design.

It may be surprising that we do not differentiate between audio and video recorders or between hand-held, low-speed, miniature, dictation tape decks and the high-speed, multi-channel tape decks associated with large computer facilities. This is because the principle of operation is the same for all tape recorders. That principle is simply moving a tape with magnetic properties by an electromagnet that is under the influence of a varying signal to make a recording. Moving the magnetized tape across another electromagnet, thereby inducing a current in the electromagnet that is then fed into an amplifier, allows for reproduction.

The Direct Tape Recorder

The major parts of a tape recorder are the system necessary to move the tape past the heads (the tape transport), the heads themselves, and the amplifiers necessary to supply the current to magnetize the tape and to generate an output signal from the pattern on the tape.

MECHANICS

The tape handling system consists of two hubs that hold the tape supply reel and a take-up reel plus the machinery necessary to pull the tape past the heads. The drive mechanism typically comprises a constant-speed motor coupled by a rubber friction drive wheel to a *capstan,* which moves the tape. The motor shaft can drive various-size wheels, thereby offering differing tape speeds. The tape is forced against the capstan by a rubber wheel called the *pinch roller.* The tape is pulled along by the capstan because it is pressed against it by the pinch roller. When the play button is pressed, the motor is energized and the pinch roller is pressed against the tape. Fig. 9-1 shows the tape path, the heads, and the drive mechanism of the tape recorder.

Early tape machines fed tape through the recorder from one reel to a second reel. For purposes of convenience, tape deck manufacturers developed cartridges to eliminate the need for an independent take-up reel. The first tape cartridge contained a single reel on which the tape was spooled in an endless loop. The tape was fed to the heads from the inside of the reel and back onto the reel from the outside. This caused the tape to slide over itself as the reel turned and thus early cartridges frequently stopped because a layer of tape stuck to the next layer of tape and wound itself too tightly. These problems were lessened by the development of lubricants of one kind or another to ease tape-sliding, but nevertheless most single-reel cartridges are now obsolete.

Current cartridges, called *cassettes,* use two reels but the entire mechanism is encased in a single shell of plastic, eliminating the inconvenience of open reel-to-reel tapes. The costs of the convenience of cartridges are that, in making smaller cartridges, manufacturers are using thinner tape (the implications of which are discussed later) and running the tape at slower speeds, which has implications for frequency response, head construction, quality of the transport mechanism, and quality of recording, as we shall see.

The quality of a tape recorder is a function of the mechanical or electrical design in its construction. In general, electrical devices are less variable in recording and reproduction quality than mechanical devices so that the more expensive the tape machine, the more likely it is to use electrical rather than mechanical components in its design where there is a choice between the two.

In those machines that might be considered for home use or for other less critical applications, the components of operation are entirely mechanical. The capstan is driven by a belt stretched between a stepped motor pulley with several different sizes and a similar stepped motor

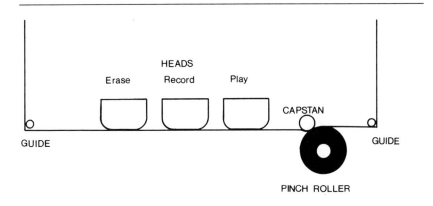

FIG. 9-1.   Tape path (represented by semirectangular border) on a direct tape recorder/reproducer.

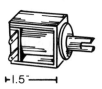

FIG. 9-2.   Type of solenoid found in tape machines.

pulley on the capstan itself. The speed of the tape can be changed by moving the belt from one set of pulleys on the motor and capstan to another set that has a different size ratio and hence a different ratio between motor speed and capstan speed. When the play button is pressed, the pinch roller is moved against the tape by a system of levers to drive the tape. The rewind and fast forward functions are also mechanically controlled by a system of gears and pulleys so that the motor can also drive the take-up and supply reels.

More expensive machines use an electromechanical system. In this case the activation of a push-button energizes devices called *solenoids*. A solenoid is an electromagnet and an attached rod that can perform mechanical operations by being attracted or repelled by the electromagnet. Fig. 9-2 is an illustration of a solenoid.

The advantage of solenoid operation is twofold. First, the button needs a much lighter touch because no mechanical function is being performed. The electrical system energizes only the solenoid, and the solenoid itself may be adjusted to determine the distance over which some mechanical linkage moves. Second, solenoid operation allows all of the functions of the tape recorder to be remotely controlled; the operator needs only a set of push-buttons that are electrically connected to sole-noids that, in turn, control the mechanical movements of the tape parts.

RECORDING ELECTRONICS

To record a signal, a source of EMF is applied to the machine from a transducer or generator. Most machines have two types of inputs: micro-phone and line. The microphone input is constructed to match the impedance of the microphone that is supplied with the machine and also to provide preamplification sufficient to boost the 100 mV or so micro-phone input to about 1 V. Most high-quality, studio-type machines will accept microphones with 50- to 250-Ω impedance, balanced. The line input is constructed so that a signal of about 1 V or more can be con-nected. Multiple inputs are sometimes available and will be briefly dis-cussed later under mixers.

Next, from the microphone or line input the signal is boosted and the electron flow is passed through a coil called the record head. The record head is actually a split-ring of one of a variety of materials, usually ferric alloys, wrapped with a coil of wire. A signal passing through the coil creates an electromagnet with lines of force that flow through the gap in the coil; these lines of force reverse direction as the polarity of the signal reverses. As the coated tape moves past the gap, it is magnetized with the various polarities that are present at the gap and with a magnetic strength that is a function of the current in the electromagnetic head. The oxide particles on the tape are magnetized in the pattern that is analogous to the flow of current through the head. In order for the op-erator to hear what is being fed into the machine, most machines have provisions for routing the input signal to the playback amplifier in addi-tion to the record amplifier. (A warning here: If one is recording through a microphone and the signal is being monitored through a loudspeaker, there is the possibility that the amplified signal from the speaker may be picked up by the microphone and then amplified again and picked up from the speaker and amplified again, and so on. If this happens, the signal continues to increase and the system will eventually begin to emit a howling noise. This is called positive feedback and can be avoided on most machines by turning off the speaker during some recording opera-tions. There is often a switch expressly for this function.)

The transfer function (i.e., the relation of input to output) of electro-magnetic devices is not linear over much of its range. Tape recorders typically use a very high frequency "bias" signal (36,000–75,000 Hz for audio) onto which the desired audio signal is superimposed. The bias signal serves to overcome some of the problems inherent in magnetizing the oxide on the tape. A complete description of the biasing process can be found in Stewart or Davies (see Suggested Reading).

THE RECORDING METER

There is an optimal current necessary for recording heads, so it is necessary both to control this current and to ensure that the optimal signal is being fed to the head. Most machines today have a meter that reads the amount of current being fed to the head and a gain control on the recording amplifier to set the level of current. Better tape recorders use a volume unit (VU) meter to monitor the level. The VU meter is a special meter whose impedance and ballistic characteristics are specified by the electronics industry. The specification of the characteristics of VU meters provides assurance that a signal recorded on one machine will play back similarly on another.

SIGNAL REPRODUCTION

The play function is essentially the opposite of the record function. The magnetized tape is passed by a coil of wire (the reproduction head) that has an EMF induced in it from the magnetic pattern on the tape. This EMF is amplified and the result is a more or less faithful copy of the original signal. The amplifier that handles this function is called the playback amplifier, which has a gain control for the output level. On inexpensive machines this control is on the same shaft as the record level control or may even be the same control. More expensive machines have separate controls, the advantage of this being that both the record and the playback levels may be set independently, each to its own optimum.

DESIGN CONSIDERATIONS

To prevent accidental erasure of a tape, tape recorders usually require something more complex than simply pressing a button to activate the record function. Many machines have a record button that must be held down while the play button is pushed. Other machines have switches that must be set or red lights that are energized when the record function is in use; some machines even have all three safeguards.

The switching for many two-head machines is shown in Fig. 9-3. Notice that the record function connects both the head to the recording amplifier and the input signal to the playback amplifier. In the play function the head is connected to the playback amplifier, and the erase head is de-energized. The same head handles the record and play functions. When one head must handle both play and record functions there are design compromises necessary so that neither record nor playback is quite optimum. More expensive machines have separate heads for each of these functions; these machines are sometimes called three-head machines. The principal advantage of a three-head machine is that the record head may be designed with sufficiently heavy wire that stronger currents may be passed through it, allowing strong signals to be im-

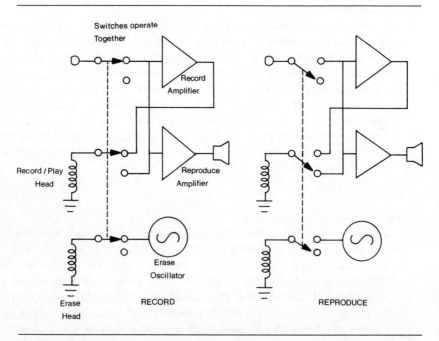

FIG. 9-3.   Switching for two-head tape machine.

pressed on the tape. The playback head may then have fine wire, but many turns of it, so that the head is very sensitive. Three-head machines also allow the operator to hear what is on the tape as it is being recorded since the tape passes first over the record head where the signal is recorded, and then over the playback head. These machines have an additional control that determines whether the playback amplifier is being fed from the input signal or the playback head and also have separate gain controls for recording and for playback.

The operation of the transport in the play mode is the same as it is in the record function because the tape moves along the same path and at the same speed as for record. When the play button is pressed, an electrical connection is made to the drive motor. On mechanical machines, this button stays in position and the electrical connection is held. In electromechanical machines, this button activates a relay that holds itself closed until a stop button is pressed. Fig. 9-4 shows a self-holding or *latching* relay schematic. When play is pressed, the relay closes and holds itself closed through its own contacts. When stop is pressed, the relay coil is de-energized and the electrical circuit opens up. On mechanically operated decks, the play button also moves the pinch roller so that the tape is pressed against the tape drive shaft, or capstan, and thus the tape is pulled through the machine and past the heads as previously discussed.

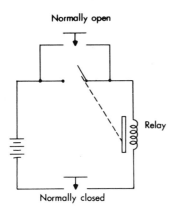

Normally open

Relay

Normally closed

FIG. 9-4.   Latching relay circuit.

To keep the tape from spilling onto the floor, the take-up reel must turn to wind the tape as it is pulled past the heads, while at the same time the supply reel must be driven in the opposite direction to maintain tension on the tape. On most inexpensive machines the same motor that feeds the tape is also connected to the take-up reel by a belt or gears. In this case, when the play button is pressed the belt is engaged and the take-up reel turns, keeping the tape under tension. On more expensive machines there is a separate motor that is energized at the same time as the drive motor through the same relay system. Because the take-up reel need supply only a slight amount of tension to the tape, the voltage supplied to this motor is less than that necessary for the motor to move at maximum speed and torque.

In the play function, the voltage is supplied through a resistor. In the fast forward function, the motor receives the full voltage so that it can spin faster and with greater torque. On mechanical machines the speed of the take-up reel is controlled by using a different size pulley from that used in the play operation. Activating the fast forward button then moves a belt to a position where it can drive the take-up reel.

In the rewind function, the less expensive machines use a mechanical system in which a belt to the drive motor engages the supply reel so that it turns at a higher rate of speed and with sufficient torque to pull the tape from the take-up reel back to the supply reel. On more expensive electromechanical machines, the rewind button activates another motor that drives only the supply reel. There are several major differences between the electromechanical and the mechanical tape transport: (1) the electromechanical machine may be remotely operated, (2) all of its functions take place following brief switch closures, while the mechanical machine is controlled by pressing buttons that stay latched, and (3) electromechanical machines usually have three motors, one each for rewind, fast forward, and play-record; an additional advantage of this, besides the elimination of the intermediate gearing and pulleys used on the single motor machine, is that if a motor performs only one function it need not be as large as those that must drive several components.

The heads are devices that put the signal on the tape and that play it back. There is also an additional head called the erase head, which removes any signal that may be on the tape, thus preparing the tape for recording. Most machines in the erase function apply a high-frequency bias to the tape, as described earlier, and because it cannot be amplified by the playback amplifier, this bias is never heard. Common values for erase signals are 48 kHz and 75 kHz. When the record button is pressed, a high-frequency oscillator is activated and feeds a signal to the erase head. This is the first head over which the tape passes.

The laws of physics that control the principles underlying tape recording specify that the faster the tape moves, the greater the signal generated in a playback head. Also, the greater the area of tape magnetized, the greater the signal. Thus, if a recording is made at 30 inches per second (ips) (i.e., 30 inches of tape move past the head every second) and on the full width of the ¼-inch tape, a stronger signal will result than if the tape is recorded at 3¾ ips and/or on ⅛-inch of the width. The early tape recorders moved the tape at a high rate to ensure a strong signal, but with the development of better heads and tapes, high speeds were no longer necessary. Also, in order to magnetize the tape at high frequencies, the tape must be moving at a higher speed than if one is recording at low frequencies. There is a minimal distance that must separate the *magnetic stripes* on the tape and if the tape is not moving fast enough to keep these separate, the signal will not be recorded. For most purposes in speech recording, 3¾ ips is sufficient.

In the early days, recording heads impressed the signal on the full width of the tape. Better heads, though, allowed the design of machines in which only half the width of the tape is recorded. Thus the tape head has only ⅛-inch of active surface. Machines with such heads are called *half-track,* as opposed to the earlier *full-track,* machines. It is possible to record on one-half the width of the tape and then pass the tape through the heads again and record on the other half of the tape. With the advent of stereophonic recording, which requires two simultaneous channels, heads that had two separate coils in them were designed. Each coil records and plays one-half the tape, requiring two of each kind of electronic component. The result is a *half-track stereo* recording. The designation of the track width has nothing to do with the number of channels that may be simultaneously recorded or played.

Later, heads were designed that record and play one-fourth the width of the tape. These are *quarter-track* tape machines. Since four channels can be recorded simultaneously, these machines are designated quarter-track, or *quadraphonic,* tape recorders. Large professional machines used in studios often have as many as 48 tracks, using, of course, tape wider than ¼ inch. These can be likened to a room filled with 48 amplifiers and speakers so that one could play a tape of a small symphony orchestra in which each artist would have a separate track on the tape.

FM Tape recording

The tape recorder found most often in the clinic and the home is a direct magnetic tape recorder. Although this recorder works on the principles previously described, its frequency response is limited by the construction of the coils in the heads and the coating on the tape. Since the changing magnetic lines of force are responsible for the magnetization of the tape, if a constant voltage level is fed to the heads there will be no movement of the lines of force and thus no magnetization of the tape. However, in some cases it is desirable to record very slowly changing signals or even DC levels; many of the electrophysiologic signals encountered in the clinic, for example, are in the frequency range of 5 to 30 Hz, which is much lower than the range of most tape recorders. Air pressures in various vocal cavities also change at very slow rates. In order to record these and other such signals, an *FM tape recorder* is used.

An FM tape recorder uses an oscillator whose output frequency is a function of the voltage being fed into it. (The resulting frequency is the carrier frequency.) If the input voltage increases, the output frequency of the oscillator increases, and vice versa. In a direct-recording tape recorder, the amplitude of the signal recorded on the tape varies. In an FM machine, the amplitude is constant, but the frequency on the tape varies as a function of the input voltage. The FM tape recorder records a signal from the oscillator that is within the range of the response of the recording and playback heads. If we assume, for example, a 10,000-Hz center frequency and if the amplitude of the input signal is 0 V, the output of the oscillator will be 10,000 Hz. If the voltage amplitude of the input signal is negative, the frequency will be less than 10,000 Hz, and if the input signal is a positive voltage, the frequency will be greater than 10,000 Hz. The tape recorder is capable of recording 10,000 Hz; when it is in the record mode this frequency is recorded. If a sine wave of 100 Hz is applied to the recorder, the signal recorded on the tape will become greater than 10,000 Hz as the sine wave goes positive and less than 10,000 Hz as the sine wave goes negative, varying in a sine fashion 100 times per second. Fig. 9-5 shows this variation.

In the playback mode, the signal may be decoded by one of several techniques that eliminate the carrier frequency and recover the voltage variation that originally caused the carrier frequency to vary. The system

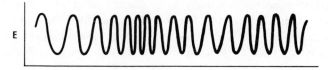

E

Time

FIG. 9-5.   Waveform generated in an FM tape machine with sine wave input.

is akin to that used in an FM radio. For a complete discussion of this the reader should refer to Langford-Smith (see Suggested Reading).

The front panel control on an FM tape recorder is similar to that on the direct recorder, but the internal adjustments are usually much more complicated. If the oscillator in the FM tape recorder changes frequency for any reason, such as aging of components or heat, the 0-V input-output frequency will be greater or less than 10,000 Hz, which will result in an output signal when there is no input signal. To compensate for this drift there is a *center frequency adjustment.* However, the clinician need not be concerned with this sort of control as long as a technician is available.

The primary drawback to the FM tape recorder is the limited frequency response due to the oscillator range and the filters necessary to decode the tape. The frequency range is also partially determined by the speed of the tape, so that most FM tape recorders have a range of speeds available to cover most of the frequencies of interest, but the response seldom covers more than a few octaves at any one speed. This is not a drawback in most electrophysiologic recording because the frequencies of interest are of limited range.

Video Tape Decks

The video tape deck is similar in principle, to the audio deck, but in operation there are two differences to be considered: first, the video signal is much more complex than the audio signal so that the video tape must receive and carry far more information, and second, the need for more information to be transmitted necessitates more complex tape transport and tape head systems.

The video receiver is, at its heart, an oscilloscope; that is, a combination of a cathode-ray gun supplying a stream of electrons and a phosphorescent screen that is illuminated when struck by a beam of electrons. The pattern that appears on the face of the tube is determined by the voltages delivered to the vertical and to the horizontal deflection plates plus the varying intensity of the beam itself. Therefore, a video deck must record and reproduce all three sets of signals (horizontal commands, vertical commands, and signal intensity).

A typical video picture is created by the beam sweeping across the screen to create a line of "dots" formed jointly by the electrons hitting the phosphorescing screen and the sawtooth wave voltage supplied to the horizontal deflection plates that progressively moves the beam from one side to the other, then returns it to begin the next line. Associated with both of these is a voltage supplied to the vertical plates that causes successive lines to appear one below another from the top to the bottom of the screen and then from the top again. This pattern of lines of dots repeated many hundreds of times per minute causes the entire screen to glow. Variation in shading at each point location is determined by the momentary intensity of the electron beam, from some maximum bright value to a momentary blanking out of the beam that results in darkness. The total image results from the repetition of a new display of dots from left to right and top to bottom many times per second.

The high rates of speed at which all three sets of commands must be delivered places great demands on the frequency response of a video tape recorder. An improved frequency response can be achieved by narrowing the gaps within the record/reproduce head(s) or by increasing tape speeds or both. The video recorder meets these stringent requirements by having the recording heads revolve clockwise past the tape, which is moving counter-clockwise. The tape is tracked so that it forms a half-circle within a circular tape guide, and the signal is applied to it by a spinning recording head that makes contact with a strip of tape that is moving in the opposite direction. Any momentary signal is placed on the tape over a distance equal to the tape speed plus the head speed. Multiple recording heads can be mounted on the rotating circle of the spinning record head assembly and spaced so that any one head delivers a signal only while a strip of unrecorded tape is in contact with it, with the next head recording the next strip, and so on.

If the tape movement is stopped while the heads continue to revolve, it is possible to reproduce the same segment of the tape repeatedly, thereby "freezing" one series of signals responsible for one video picture without tape movement. If the tape movement is reduced in speed, slow-motion reproduction is possible. In the case of freezing the motion of the reproduction, there would be no audio reproduction because the tape is not moving past the audio head; in the case of slow-motion reproduction, the audio reproduction would be frequency-shifted downward by a proportion equal to the proportion of the tape slow-down (i.e., a tape speed one-third of normal would shift all audio frequencies to one-third their normal values and stretch out the audio signal to three times its normal duration).

Digital recording techniques have been available for several years for computers, but have been adapted only recently to audio signals. The

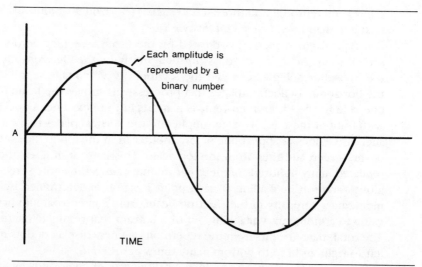

FIG. 9-6.   Digital sampling of a sine wave.

equipment is very expensive but promises excellent fidelity with no residual noise. (The latter is sometimes an unnerving experience for first-time listeners.) Digital recording works by feeding an input signal through an analog-to-digital (A/D) converter, then recording the signal as a series of pulses. On playback, the pulses are played back from the tape through a digital-to-analog (D/A) converter. The A/D converter operates by increasing the amplitude of the input signal and converting each sample amplitude to a value represented by a series of eight bits, each bit being either a one or a zero (256 different amplitude steps can be represented by eight bits, that is, 2^8 steps). Fig. 9-6 illustrates this operation. The sample time depends on the rate at which the electronics of the recorder feed the input signal to an integrated circuit (IC) that essentially measures the signal's amplitude and converts the value to a binary number that represents one of the 256 amplitude steps. The binary number is recorded on the tape. On playback, the IC changes the binary number to a voltage value equivalent to the binary number. The signal is fed through a filtering circuit that "smoothes" the step-like variations back into a continuous waveform. The principal advantage of a digital recorder is the fact that the tape retains only a series of pulses representing the amplitude. Any noise on the tape is not a part of the playback process unless it changes the value of the binary number; there can be no distortion because the signal that is recorded is a series of pulses representing numbers. The value of this number changes with input level, and, as long as the correct numerical value is repeated on playback, there can be no distortion of the amplitude.

At the present time, there are one or two self-contained digital-recording machines and several devices that adapt a video recorder for digital audio recording.

Speech Compression and Speech Expansion Systems

Audio speech compressors and speech expansion systems (speech stretchers) accomplish their tasks by using rotating audio reproduction heads, much like those in video decks. In the case of speech compression, the multi-head rotating pick-up spins in the same direction that the tape moves. Some small segment of tape is reproduced and the next small segment is omitted, but, because the reproduction head assembly moves with the tape, the reproduced portions occur without intermediate silences and the result is compressed speech.

Speech expansion is accomplished by rotating the reproduction head assembly against the direction of tape movement. In this case each small section of tape is reproduced more than one time and the rate of repetition determines the percentage of speech expansion.

Delayed Auditory Feedback

Delayed auditory feedback (DAF) is an interesting application of the principles of tape recording. Several authorities have found DAF a useful tool in therapy with those who stutter and have also used it to demonstrate the importance of auditory feedback in speech. In this technique, a signal is recorded and played back through headphones. The signal played back is delayed by an amount of time equal to the time it takes the tape to move from the record head to the playback head (i.e., a combination of distance between the heads and tape speed). Fig. 9-7 should make this clear. Note that the person speaks into the microphone and the signal is routed to the record head. The signal is recorded and the tape moves to the playback head. The signal is then taken from the head, amplified, and fed to the headphones the person who is speaking is wearing.

Commercial delayed feedback systems sometimes adapt standard recorders for this function, while others are designed for use only as delay devices. The former type has the playback head mounted on a track so it can be moved closer to or farther from the record head, thus decreasing or increasing the delay. The machine designed specifically for DAF purposes uses a tape loop and has many refinements not found in machines that are adapted for this purpose (Fig. 9-8).

The DAF tape recorder controls are of a type common to any audio

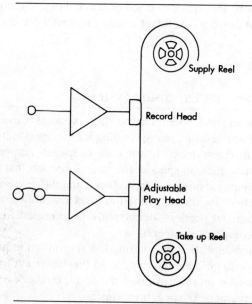

FIG. 9-7. Schematic of delayed auditory feedback tape system.

machine. There is a record gain control and either a meter or a lamp to indicate proper record level. There is also an output gain control. These usually are the extent of the controls, but the adapted machine may contain tone controls and a function selector switch. It is recommended that the tone control be set so that the output has no filtering; the output should be no different from the input. Machines designed specifically for DAF usually have provisions for one, two, or three fixed amounts of delay. The adapted machines have a head that may be moved to an infinite number of intermediate positions, a useful function for research purposes but perhaps not very important for clinical purposes.

Devices called *digital delay lines* or *"bucket brigades"* have been developed recently. These seem to be readily adaptable to delayed auditory feedback and perform this function without using tape; they are also very small, which allows the delayed auditory feedback unit to be housed in a case not much larger than a cigarette case. These DAF machines do not allow an adjustment of delay time, but this is not likely to be a problem in therapeutic applications. Such units operate by delaying the audio signal in a series of integrated circuits passing from one to another in a finite and remotely controlled time. The circuits are quite reliable and should not require maintenance, but if they do, the clinician will have to rely on an electronics technician to repair them. Fig. 9-9 illustrates a current model DAF machine that can easily be worn all day.

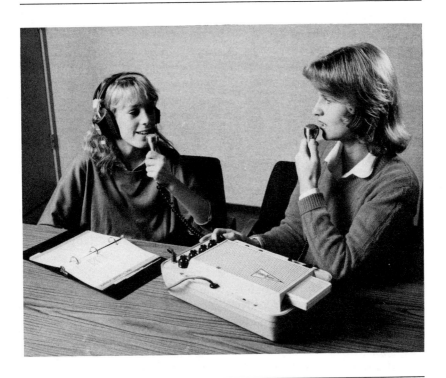

FIG. 9-8.   A tape-loop delayed auditory feedback unit for clinical use. (Courtesy Phonic Ear, HC Electronics, Inc.)

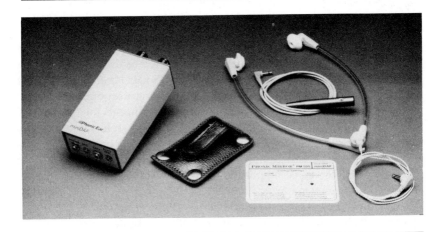

FIG. 9-9.   A small, wearable electronic delayed auditory feedback unit. (Courtesy Phonic Ear, HC Electronics, Inc.)

Recording Tape

There are two types of recording tape in use today. The less expensive is *polyester plastic* tape. This tape tends to get brittle with age, dries out quickly, and, if stored for long periods of time, even falls apart. The newer and now almost the only commonly available tape is Mylar. This tape holds oxide well (e.g., the oxide coating does not rub off readily) and does not dry out or get brittle. The only problem with Mylar is its ability to stretch. If the tape becomes entangled, it will stretch instead of breaking, which renders useless the affected section of the recording. Plastic, on the other hand, will snap cleanly so that it is a simple matter to splice the tape back together by joining the two ends and applying a piece of splicing tape.

Because the pattern on the tape is a result of magnetizing small oxide particles on the tape, the smoothness or completeness of the tape's oxide covering is important. Spots on the tape that have no oxide particles will not be magnetized. These spots are called *drop outs* and are especially detrimental for computers, where one blank spot on the tape can derail an entire program. Also, if there are spots on the tape that have a great deal of oxide, there is a strong possibility that a signal will be impressed that is very strong as compared to the signals impressed at other places on the tape. The smaller the particles, the better the high-frequency response, too. Therefore, the ideal tape has equal density and particle size throughout its length. Tapes are made in various grades of density and smoothness and are often labeled as such. Tape with a very accurate deposit is called *high-density* or sometimes *Dynarange,* a 3M trademark.

Early recording tape consisted of ferric oxide particles on a plastic base, but modern tapes are made with many different oxides, including chromium dioxide. The result is a finer particle base for smoother signal recording and a much greater magnetic level.

Tape usually cannot retain a small signal; there is a minimal level above which recording can take place. For this reason, the tape has a bias signal introduced that raises the magnetic signal fed to the tape. This bias signal is usually of a very high frequency (45–75 kHz) that is not audible, and the input signal "rides" on this. Each type of tape requires a different level of bias, and the machine should either be adjusted for the type of tape or, as some modern machines do, have a switch-selectable bias value.

A recording head records a tape by introducing both positive and negative magnetic variation, where the amount of magnetism induced is determined by signal amplitude, and the direction or polarity of the induced magnetism is a function of the polarity of the signal. If, for example, one wishes to record a 15,000-Hz tone on tape running at 10 ips, each inch of tape would have 3,000 magnetic reversals on it. If one is trying to magnetize particles with 30,000 reversals per second, the particles must be sufficiently small to allow this. If the particles are so large that they take up too much room on the tape, it will not be possible to impress such a high frequency on the tape.

For high-quality recordings that are to be stored for long periods of time (more than 2 or 3 months), it is best to use 1.5-mil (1 mil = 1/1,000 inch), Mylar, or a high-density tape. Tapes should be stored in metal cans to protect them from becoming magnetized by stray magnetic fields like those from fluorescent lights and motors. Also, stray fields tend to accelerate print-through, which is discussed in the next section. Tapes should be kept cool as heat will also cause print-through.

Another variable in recording tape is its thickness. When tape recording first became popular, the reels were 5 inches in diameter and contained about 500 feet of tape that was 1.5 mils thick. For short recordings, this appeared to be a sufficient amount of tape, but recordings of more than 15 minutes required the operator to change tapes. Because of this, manufacturers began to make the tape thinner and put more of it on a reel. The standard reel became 7 inches in diameter and contained 1,200 feet of tape. Because it allowed 1,800 feet to be put on a reel, 1-mil tape became popular. However, this caused a problem. When a tape is recorded, a magnetic pattern is put onto tape, layers of which are then wound one over the other. This means that each layer of tape is sandwiched between two other layers, each of which has a magnetic pattern on it. If the tape is sufficiently thin, the pattern on one layer can be impressed onto the layer of tape above or below it. The result is called *echo* and *pre-echo* or, more aptly, *print-through*. (Pre-echo is the faint sound of what is to come.) To avoid this, a thicker tape is used, thus separating the layers of magnetic recording by a greater distance. The maximum thickness of tape commonly available is 1.5 mils and is often labeled "low print" tape.

Tape Recorder Maintenance

HEAD-CLEANING

As the tape passes over any surface, some of the oxide becomes powdered and sticks to the heads and post over which it has passed. This oxide should be removed by dipping a cotton swab in alcohol and cleaning any surface the tape touches, including the pinch roller. The process should then be repeated using a dry swab to remove any remaining alcohol. It is very important to remove all alcohol quickly from any rubber surface such as the pinch roller since alcohol tends to dry out rubber, causing it to crack.

HEAD DEMAGNETIZATION

The heads may sometimes have static magnetic patterns that have built up due to tape moving across them. To remove this build-up, a strong magnetic field is placed close to the head by means of a coil wrapped around a soft iron pole. This AC field is gradually moved away so that it becomes weaker and weaker. Recently there has been some controversy concerning the necessity of head demagnetization, but, even if it is performed incorrectly, no harm is done if one is careful. The result of the process is that the head has a decreasing field impressed on it and eventually, when the head demagnetizer is sufficiently far away, no magnetic pattern is left. Head demagnetizers may be purchased almost anywhere tape machines are sold. The tape transport should be cleaned and the heads demagnetized every 4 to 6 hours of use.

HEAD ALIGNMENT

A frequently occurring problem with tape recorders is related to head alignment. As we have previously stated, the gap in the recording head is the point at which the magnetic field is most concentrated and hence the point at which the tape will be magnetized. If the gap is perpendicular to the path of the tape, a short pulse might appear as a minute magnetic stripe in the width of the tape. On playback this magnetic stripe passes the gap in the play head and causes an output signal to be induced in the head, but if the gap on the play head is not at the same angle as the stripe, less signal will be received at each instant in time as compared to the recording. This occurs most often when tapes are recorded on one machine and played back on another.

Thus, head alignment must be adjusted to ensure that the record and play head gaps are perpendicular to the tape path. Otherwise, a loss of high frequencies results because high frequencies produce the narrowest stripes on the tape and, therefore, are more prone to being lost in misaligned playback.

To align the play head, standard alignment tape is played, which consists of 7- to 15-kHz tones that are very carefully recorded with very precisely aligned heads. These tapes are available from various audio dealers. While this tape is being played, one of the screws that hold the play head in place is carefully adjusted for maximum output. (It is best to make certain that the screwdriver blade has not become magnetized since this may add a signal to the tape or even erase portions of it. Screwdrivers in the laboratory have a tendency to become magnetized when used around electronic equipment; one can verify that a screwdriver is not magnetized by using a tape demagnetizer on it.) If the machine has only two heads, the alignment is then complete because the erase head is not affected by small amounts of misalignment. If there is a separate record head, then a high-frequency signal is fed into the machine and the output of the tape is monitored while recording. The record head can then be adjusted for maximum output.

Head alignment may not be a job most clinicians will want to tackle, but playing an alignment tape can indicate whether head alignment is necessary, since alignment tapes have signals from 50 to 20 kHz all recorded at the same level following the 15-kHz signal. The clinician can play the tape and measure the output; if it decreases by more than about 3 dB at 10 kHz, alignment should be considered. Higher frequencies are not usually important in speech recording, and some machines, even when newly aligned, may not be capable of reproducing them.

Tape Storage

Most clinicians will have acquired a library of tapes after a short time, and, if the tapes are important, some care is necessary in their storage. To begin with, it is best if tapes can be stored in steel cases since steel prevents stray magnetic fields from erasing tapes. Film cans are excellent for 7-inch reels, whereas cassettes might best be kept in a cash box. A cool storage place is also desirable since heat can accelerate tape deterioration and print-through. If the tape is nylon or of a similar material, humidity is a problem.

Keep tapes away from motors, air conditioners, and other sources of energy consumption. Never place tapes on television sets since televisions generate strong high-frequency signals. These signals are usually confined within the television cabinet, but there may be leaks.

For especially valuable recordings it is best to not rewind the tape since the tape layers will then be looser and not in such close proximity, lessening chances of print-through. In addition, be sure to place labels on all your tapes. It is amazing how quickly we forget.

Finally, splice broken tapes only with material made for that purpose. *Never* splice recording tapes with Scotch or similar cellophane tapes. It is frightening what a layer of rubber cement can do to the fidelity of a tape transport.

Suggested Reading

Davies, G. L. *Magnetic Tape Instrumentation.* New York: McGraw-Hill, 1961.

Langford-Smith, F. *Radiotron Designer's Handbook.* Harrison, N.J.: RCA, 1953.

Malmstadt, H. V., and Enke, C. G. *Electronics for Scientists.* New York: Benjamin, 1963.

Malmstadt, H. V., and Enke, C. G. *Digital Electronics for Scientists.* New York: Benjamin, 1969.

Stewart, W. E. *Magnetic Recording Techniques.* New York: McGraw-Hill, 1958.

10. Signal Generators

The term *signal generator* is used to specify equipment that provides an AC signal of a selected amplitude and waveshape. There are two general types of instruments for performing signal generation: the oscillator and the function generator.

Oscillators

We may say that, in general, the *oscillator* is a device for producing sine waves of selectable frequency and amplitude. The most common method of producing sine waves makes use of tuned circuits of coils, capacitors, and resistors as elements in the feedback of an operational amplifier. (Operational amplifiers were discussed in detail in Chap. 4.) Because the gain of the operational amplifier varies as a function of the feedback elements, if the feedback elements are frequency dependent (i.e., the gain of the amplifier is very large at the resonant frequency and practically zero at any other), the result is an oscillator. Almost all modern oscillators use some variation of this general theme to generate sine waves. The accuracy of the frequency output of this type of oscillator will be a function of the accuracy of the feedback (tunable) elements, so it is necessary to monitor the signal carefully if frequency is an important variable. Once an oscillator has been adjusted and the variation of the circuit elements accounted for, the principal culprit leading to error in the output frequency is the power supply. The power supply must be very carefully designed and stabilized because changes in power-supply voltage can lead to changes in the tuning of the feedback elements.

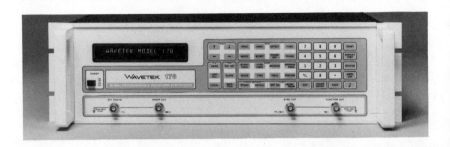

FIG. 10-1.   Modern programmable waveform/frequency synthesizer. (Courtesy Wavetek San Diego, Inc., San Diego.)

A method of generating sine waves that is easy to calibrate uses an instrument called a *beat-frequency oscillator* (BFO). The BFO consists of two oscillators, one fixed and the other variable, whose outputs are combined in a network in which the output frequency is equal to the difference in frequency between the two generators in the instrument. The dial of the BFO has a zero point, and at this point the frequencies of the fixed and variable oscillators are equal. The instrument has in series with the main tuning control, a small control that allows the operator to adjust the frequency of the variable oscillator so that it equals the frequency of the fixed oscillator. The main tuning control dial is set to the zero point. The machine can be calibrated by following these steps: establishment of the zero point is ensured once there is no output from the device (no output is possible at zero frequency because zero frequency is not an AC signal). To select any other frequency, one of the oscillators is tuned by a front panel control labeled *output frequency* (or something similar). The tunable oscillator is constructed to be adjustable, but with very stable output.

There are several basic designs used in oscillators. *Wein Bridge oscillators* are the most common, least expensive, and typically least adequate signal generators because of their variability. Beat frequency oscillators are more expensive than Wein Bridge oscillators, provide pure sine waves, and can cover the entire audio range with one sweep of the dial. They can also be calibrated very easily. The third type of generator, *frequency synthesizers,* provide accurate frequencies and may also be programmed (i.e., controlled) by a computer or a similar device.

Frequency synthesizers, which are modern sine wave generators, make use of integrated circuits called *phase-locked loops* that have a variety of uses. Phase-locked loops are rather complex but can generate precise signals whose frequencies can be selected by switching in various resistive and reactive elements. The face of one modern frequency synthesizer is shown in Fig. 10-1. Note that there is simply a series of push-buttons that can be activated to select any frequency within the range of the instrument with an accuracy of one cycle. This type of tuning obviously eliminates the inaccuracies of tuning dials and the extrapolation associated with tuning dials. Finally, the phase-locked circuit can also be incorporated into a device that can interface with a computer in such a way that the output part of the computer need only supply a binary number to the synthesizer. Switches within the synthesizer tune to the frequency specified by a particular combination of zeros and ones. Larger computers, which are discussed in Chapter 14, need not have the addition of the synthesizer since they are capable of generating any waveform by a series of binary numbers that approximate the shape of any wave desired.

Function Generators

Another type of signal generator is called a *function generator*. This device often provides sine, square, and sawtooth waves. Still other generators provide a sweep frequency output, which will be discussed shortly.

A square wave, having an appearance of a square-cornered wave, contains a fundamental frequency and all of the odd harmonics of the fundamental. The sawtooth wave (discussed in Chap. 8) contains the fundamental and all of the harmonics and is important to speech research because the glottal waveform resembles a sawtooth. The function generator delivers a sawtooth into a series of filters representing the vocal tract to recreate vowels and, with the proper switching, some consonants. The function generator can also be used to provide calibration signals for the sound spectrograph by supplying a signal with many harmonics so that an unknown signal can be duplicated and thus its frequency determined as in analysis-by-synthesis.

A *tone burst* from a signal generator is an output that is present only when a specified voltage input level is exceeded at the trigger input. This tone burst consists of a controllable number of cycles of the signal. A unit with tone burst is of more value to the psychoacoustician than to the speech researcher.

The secret of the function generator's ability to produce waves other than sine waves is a series of circuits that change the basic sine wave into other types of signals. As an example, consider infinite peak-clipping of a sine wave. If the tops of a train of sine waves are progressively clipped and subsequently amplified, the resulting wave approaches a square wave shape. Newer signal generators make use of integrated circuit chips to perform the wave-shaping. To generate square waves, a circuit called an *astable multivibrator* may be used. This is simply a pair of semiconductor devices in which one or the other circuit is turned on: one provides a positive voltage and the other a negative. The result is an output that

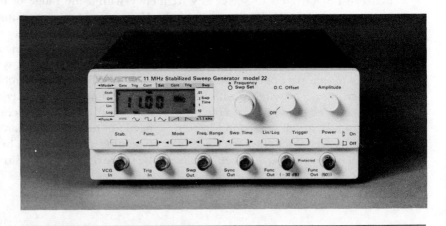

FIG. 10-2.   Function sweep generator with digital readout. (Courtesy Wavetek San Diego, Inc., San Diego.)

consists of alternate periods of positive and negative voltage of fixed value and nothing in between.

To generate triangular waves, a square wave going only positively is fed into an integrator. Since the voltage seen by the integrator will be constant, the integrator will show a linear increase in voltage until the square wave switches to zero, at which point the output will linearly decrease. To generate a sawtooth wave a similar arrangement is used (but in this case the integrator looks at some constant positive value of voltage). When the integrator reaches some specified value going in the positive direction, a switching circuit discharges the integrator capacitor and the value drops, instantaneously, to zero. Then integration begins again.

Fig. 10-2 is an example of the front panel of a function generator. The frequency knob is immediately to the right of the digital readout and determines the frequency output of the unit.

In many cases, there is a "multiplier" switch, which multiplies the frequency selected by a frequency dial. If, for example, the frequency dial is at 1.0 and the multiplier is at 1,000, the nominal reading of the frequency dial is to be multiplied by 1,000, and, in this example, the output is 1,000 Hz.

The BFO is one signal generator that does not usually require a multiplier because the central dial can cover the entire range of frequencies. A single dial sweeping the entire range of frequencies is not always desirable since it limits the accuracy to which one may set the frequency without a meter. In some circumstances, however, as with the Békésy audiometer, one dial is preferable.

In Fig. 10-2, the output plug is at the right and consists of a BNC connector (connectors are discussed in Chap. 15). Below the digital readout is a display of the kind of waveform generated. The small knob at the upper right is the amplitude control, which is used to determine the amplitude of the signal but is not calibrated. Some oscillators and function generators have a continuous control and a switch labeled in decibels. The control varies the amplitude of the signal continuously and the switch attenuates it in 10-dB steps. The 10-dB step switch is a useful feature, but remember that the decibel markings on this dial do not bear any relationship to decibel sound pressure level or hearing threshold. The decibel relationship holds only between various steps on the switch.

Most function generators have a low-output impedance so that they will not alter the operation of the circuit to which they are connected. If they are connected into a circuit that alters their operation, they may or may not function as generators, but they will not function accurately in any case. Common output impedance values are 500 Ω and 50 Ω. If audiometric headphones are connected directly to an oscillator they will not operate very effectively because of their 10-Ω impedance. Also, most attenuators are 500/600-Ω units, and the attenuator dials are only accurate if their sources and loads are between 500- and 600-Ω impedance. An attenuator can be used with a different input impedance if an impedance-matching transformer is imposed or if 25 to 30 dB of attenuation is inserted constantly. That is, the circuit is adjusted with the attenuator dials set between 25 and 30 dB to begin with, and the system is calibrated with this amount of attenuation or more in the circuit, to prevent the mismatched impedance from altering the frequency characteristics of the circuit.

Some function generators, especially *voltage-controlled generators* (VCGs), offer a "sweep frequency" output. The VCG is an instrument containing elements such that the output frequency is a function of the voltage applied to the input (see Chap. 9). Precise control of the input voltage allows equally precise control over the output frequency. Oscillators are available with a front panel input and control so that the frequency of the output can be controlled by an external input voltage. The generator shown in Fig. 10-2 is constructed to offer VCG operation. The external voltage input is shown on the left side of the unit. The tuning of the VCG is accomplished by using reactive elements whose reactances vary as a function of an applied voltage.

To obtain a sweep output from a VCG, a sawtooth (ramp) input voltage is connected to the control unit. The ramp voltage appears as in Fig. 10.3. The ramp voltage increases linearly from some minimal value that determines the lowest frequency generated to some maximum voltage and frequency output, and then drops back to the initial voltage. The voltage causes the output frequency to increase at a constant rate and then drop back to its initial value. The result is a sweep frequency output. This type

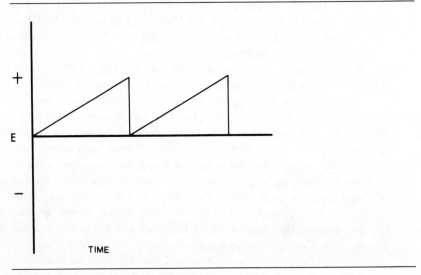

FIG. 10-3.   Ramp voltage waveform.

of signal is very useful in aligning filters or in testing the bandwidth of a circuit.

The most important factor for the speech researcher to bear in mind in selecting a signal generator is the sensitivity of the auditory system. The human subject is highly sensitive to variations in amplitude in the signal generator, so that any sound source providing a presumably constant amplitude output must meet rigorous quality standards. Otherwise, variations in signal generator output may obscure the experimental result sought in the study. For example, the type of instrument in use in the radio and television service shop is seldom adequate for speech research.

Suggested Reading

Hoagland, A. A.   *Digital Magnetic Recording.* Melbourne, Fla.: Krieger, 1983.
Rettinger, M.   *Practical Electroacoustics.* New York: Chemical Publishing, 1955.

IV. Equipment Evaluation

IV. Equipment Evaluation

11. Amplifiers, Microphones, and Loudspeakers

Equipment evaluation requires examining the same few parameters (e.g., frequency response, signal-to-noise ratio) that have been considered previously, plus some characteristics that are of special concern for each type of equipment. The reader will profit by examining the performance of each of the most common types of equipment individually, although an overview of the analysis procedures will reveal that there are only a few basic building blocks from which almost any sort of processor can be constructed.

Techniques for Evaluating Amplifiers

Many electronic characteristics are important in evaluating an amplifier, but four are most often specified. They are frequency response (or frequency distortion), signal-to-noise ratio, sensitivity, and nonlinear distortion (most commonly, amplitude distortion).

FREQUENCY DISTORTION

Frequency distortion occurs when a device does not process all frequencies equally. Distortion is most evident as peaks and troughs in a graph of the output amplitude versus frequency (the transfer function), when the input is a constant-amplitude, frequency-varying signal; this graph is the frequency-response curve. The simplest method for measuring frequency response consists of feeding an oscillator signal into the amplifier, measuring the output, and then changing the frequency and measuring

177

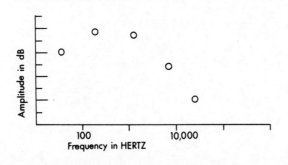

FIG. 11-1.   Frequency-response chart.

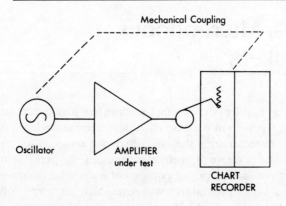

FIG. 11-2.   Automatic frequency-response plotting equipment.

the output again, continuing this operation so as to assess the entire range of frequencies. The output measurements are recorded on a chart, with frequency on the abscissa and the amplitude, usually expressed in volts or decibels, on the ordinate. Fig. 11-1 shows an example of a frequency-response measurement. Of course, the operator would make certain that the input to the amplifier is a constant value as the frequency is changed. This technique can be time consuming and tedious, so more rapid and efficient automatic methods have been developed.

In the automatic methods of measuring the frequency response of an amplifier, an oscillator whose frequency control is driven by a motor is connected to the amplifier input. The output of the amplifier is connected to a graphic level recorder. The level recorder paper chart is driven by the same motor as the oscillator. Fig. 11-2 is a block diagram of the arrangement. To measure frequency response, the level recorder uses paper charts that have amplitude and frequency coordinates. The oscil-

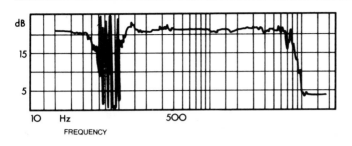

FIG. 11-3.   Chart from automatic response system.

lator is set at the lower end of the frequency range, the paper chart is positioned so that the same frequency is under the pen, and the motor is started. The oscillator sweeps through the range and the chart moves in synchrony. The final result might appear as in Fig. 11-3.

Several precautionary steps are important in the automatic measuring system. First, the oscillator output voltage should be relatively constant. Almost any oscillator can maintain an output of + 0.1 dB, which is adequate for measuring almost any amplifier. Second, the amplifier must have the proper load impedance connected at its output. If one is measuring a power amplifier the load is usually 4 to 16 Ω. A resistor is best as a load, rather than a loudspeaker, for example, since the loudspeaker will not have a constant impedance because it embodies reactance. The result is that under a speaker load the amplifier will have a varying load, which may cause amplitude variations. (It is important to remember that the output may be several watts, so sufficiently large resistors should be connected.) Of course, if one is evaluating an entire amplifier-speaker system, then the speaker will have to remain connected. Third, the response of the amplifier may vary, depending on the level at which it is driven. Power amplifiers are conventionally measured with their outputs set at 1 W or at half power or at full power. Individual laboratories use other levels, but if only one level is chosen, the half-power point is a good compromise since with music and speech the output seldom exceeds this level for longer than fractions of a second. As a matter of fact, the average power output of most home music systems is less than 1 W.

There is no standard method for rating amplifiers in terms of frequency response; the chart of the response is simply published (for example, the Index of Response Irregularity in Jerger [see Suggested Reading]). Certainly an amplifier for speech exhibits a response of ± 1 dB from 50 Hz to 15 kHz would be adequate. For special amplifiers the frequency range may be much different. Electrophysiologic amplifiers, for instance, often have to extend down to less than 1 Hz, or even DC (0 Hz), and seldom have to extend above 2,000 Hz. Again, there are no data that would support a more rigid criterion than $\pm$ 1 dB unless the amplifier is to be used in psychoacoustic studies in which $\pm$ 0.25 dB is about the limit of resolving power of the auditory nerve.

SIGNAL-TO-NOISE RATIO

Signal-to-noise ratio (S/N) is the ratio of the output voltage, with all the controls at their maximum, to the output where there is no signal input. In practice, an oscillator is connected to the input of the amplifier and the voltage across the output load is measured at some midband frequency (often 1,000 Hz). Then the input to the amplifier is shorted to ground and the output measured again. The decibel equation

$$dB = 20 \log \frac{V_{out} \text{ normal}}{V_{out} \text{ shorted in}}$$

yields a dB value for the S/N. Most amplifiers will exhibit at least 70 dB, and even 80 dB would be desirable for most applications. Again, there is no standardized measuring technique or criterion.

SENSITIVITY

Sensitivity is a measure of the input signal necessary to obtain the maximum rated output of the amplifier. This is measured by applying an input signal, usually at 400 or 1,000 Hz, and monitoring the output signal until it reaches the maximum rated value. The value of the input signal is then measured and is used as an indicator of the sensitivity.

Amplifier components, like elements of other equipment, are designed to operate with reasonable fidelity, but they typically will do so only within a limited range. Therefore, one facet of characterizing amplifiers is to designate the range within which the amplifier will deliver specified performance. For example, the input of an amplifier for use in electromyographic measurement must work with 10 μV (0.000010 V), while the output of an audio amplifier for a high-fidelity system may be working in the range of 100 V. The audio output is thus 10,000,000, or 10^7, times greater than the electromyographic input. These widely varying needs result in quite different requirements (e.g., the allowable noise level in an amplifier that is to reproduce faithfully a signal in the microvolt or nanovolt range is infinitesimal compared to the acceptable noise level of an audio power amplifier) and necessitate technical specifications of minimum and maximum signal levels as well as maximum noise levels for each type of amplifier.

AMPLITUDE DISTORTION

Amplitude distortion is any distortion that causes a change in the shape of the waveform between the input and the output. There are several common distortion measurements, but we will limit our discussion to

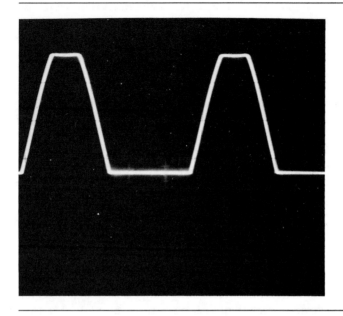

FIG. 11-4.   A sine wave that has been subjected to severe peak clipping.

harmonic distortion and intermodulation distortion. These two types of distortion are termed *nonlinear* because they are the result of an amplifier process that is not linear between input and output.

Harmonic Distortion

To explain harmonic distortion, consider a sine wave fed to an amplifier with some gain. The output should be simply an increased amplitude of the sine wave. If the amplifier cannot amplify all of the signal input, however, the output might appear as in Fig. 11-4. The peaks of the sine waves have been clipped off. The amplifier could only amplify the sine wave over a portion of a cycle and was unable to continue amplifying at the peaks—the amplifier is *overloaded,* and the result is *peak-clipping.* Peak-clipping results in the generation of odd harmonics of the input frequency.

There are two principal methods for measuring harmonic distortion. In one method a sine wave is fed in and the output voltage is measured. Then the output signal is passed through a reflection filter tuned to the input signal. A rejection filter allows all frequencies to pass except the narrow band to which it is tuned. The output voltage is measured again, and the result is an indication of the amount of signal that is at frequencies other than the input. The percentage of the total output (without the rejection filter) represented by the distortion products (with the rejection filter) is called *total harmonic distortion* (THD).

The second method of measuring harmonic distortion, which is specified for hearing aids, uses a sine wave input, but a narrow bandpass filter is used in measuring the output. The sine wave is fed in, the output is measured, and then the output is fed through the filter. The filter is tuned to each harmonic of the input signal, and the output at each harmonic is measured. The total amount of harmonic distortion measured by this method consists of the percentage of the total output represented by the *sum* of all of the harmonics. A wave analyzer can also be used to obtain a distortion measure. Recall from Chapter 2 that a wave analyzer will display the frequency composition of a signal fed into it. Therefore, if the output of the amplifier under test is displayed on a wave analyzer, it is possible to extract voltage values for each harmonic without the necessity of tuning an individual filter.

Harmonic distortion values of 0.1% are common and probably acceptable for most power amplifiers. Bear in mind that 0.1% distortion can be translated as 1/1,000 of the total output and that one part in a thousand parts of voltage is equal to -60 dB. This means that the harmonics are only 60 dB below the fundamental.

Harmonic distortion measurement techniques have been specified for a variety of devices, including hearing aids (ANSI S3.3-1971 [R1960]) and audiometers (ANSI S3.6-1969 [R1973]). An input frequency of 400 Hz is commonly used in broadcast equipment, and a series of frequencies is specified for hearing aids. Distortion is often measured at 1-W, half-power, and maximum-power outputs.

There are specialized distortion-measuring instruments that will continuously measure the distortion as the amplitude of the input signal is varied, with the frequency held constant, or as the frequency is varied, with the amplitude held constant.

Intermodulation Distortion

Intermodulation distortion measurement is another method of specifying amplitude distortion and is based on the premise that signals in amplifiers consist of more than simple sine waves and that there can be some interaction between components of complex signals. The measurement is made by feeding two sine waves, one of low frequency and one of high frequency, to the amplifier. The lower frequency (F_L) has a voltage four times that of the higher frequency (F_H). The rationale for this is that in most speech and music signals there will be much more low-frequency energy than there is at high frequencies. Usual frequencies are 400 Hz for the lower frequency and 1,250 Hz for the higher frequency (values that are not harmonically related must be chosen).

If the amplifier has nonlinear distortion, the output will consist of the input frequencies and also the sum and difference frequencies. That is, the output could be 400 Hz (F_L), 1,250 Hz (F_H), 850 Hz ($F_H - F_L$), or 1,650 Hz ($F_H + F_L$). The output could even consist of sums and differences of harmonics: 450 Hz ($F_H - 2 F_L$), 50 Hz ($F_H - 3 F_L$), 2,100 Hz ($2 F_H - F_L$), and so on. In any case, the output voltage of the amplifier is measured, and then the output is fed to an analyzer that measures these sums and differences, either individually or in total.

These general guidelines can be followed in evaluating almost any device containing amplifiers, with some obvious modifications of the techniques. For example, if one were to assess the quality of a root-mean-square voltmeter, the frequency response measurement might be important. The necessary modification would be that the output would be read on the voltmeter itself. Or, to assess a filter, there would be no change in the frequency response technique because the frequency response is the criterion of interest.

Techniques for Evaluating Microphones

There are several important specifications used in selecting a microphone, including frequency response, directional characteristics, and sensitivity. Microphone evaluation must be performed in a sound-isolated environment because the microphone will transduce all acoustic signals, not just the test signals, and extraneous signals can obviously contaminate the measures. Microphone manufacturers use double-walled anechoic chambers. An *anechoic chamber* is a room in which the walls are covered with materials so that there is no sound reflection from the walls. The signal fed directly to the microphone from the speaker is the only signal of interest; reflected signals will only obfuscate the accuracy of the microphone output. If a sound-isolated room without reflectors is not available, it is possible to make measurements late at night (when it is relatively quiet) in an open area outdoors (to prevent reflections).

FREQUENCY RESPONSE

A frequency response is a measurement of how well the microphone responds to varying frequencies. To test this, the microphone is placed in a sound field in which the frequency is varied, but the amplitude of the signal is held constant or readjusted at each frequency to some constant value. The output of the microphone is recorded at the various frequencies, usually using a voltmeter.

This technique is comparable to the amplifier technique, but there is a major confounding problem with assessing microphones: the acoustic signal, which is the input to the microphones, must be constant regardless of frequency, and loudspeakers seldom exhibit flat, broadband response. For this reason, it is necessary to measure the acoustic output of the speaker to make certain it is constant. This means that a high-quality microphone of sufficiently flat response is placed next to the microphone

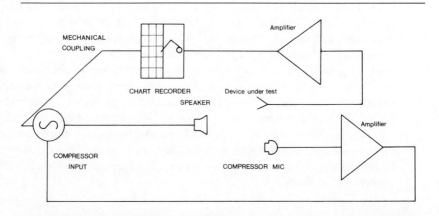

FIG. 11-5.   Block diagram of automatic response plotter with compressor. MIC = microphone.

under test. Then, as the frequency to the loudspeaker is changed, the acoustic output is adjusted to the chosen value. Often a microphone is measured at 70 to 80 dB because this sound pressure level approximates speech levels. The technique just described is even more cumbersome than for measuring amplifiers, so an automatic method has been developed.

In the automatic method of measuring the frequency response of a microphone, it is desirable that the input to the microphone be of a constant level so that variations in the microphone output express only the variations in the sensitivity of the microphone itself. Most often, however, the acoustic signal is presented by a small loudspeaker that may not itself have a flat frequency response. To correct the fluctuations in output of the speaker (i.e., the input to the microphone), a feedback system from the loudspeaker output to the oscillator controlling its input is added to allow for variations in response of the output system. Fig. 11-5 shows the basic circuit. The *compressor input* to the oscillator is a special electrical circuit controlling the output of the oscillator as a function of an input signal at the compressor input. If the voltage input is large, the output of the oscillator is small. If the compressor input decreases, the output of the oscillator increases and vice versa. A microphone with an extremely good (i.e., flat) frequency response is connected to this input and is placed in front of the loudspeaker. If the output of the speaker increases, the input to the compressor will increase, which will cause the output of the oscillator to decrease. With a smaller output from the oscillator, the loudspeaker will produce less, so the microphone will receive less, and cause the compressor input to decrease and the output of the oscillator to increase. That is, the output of the speaker is used to alter the

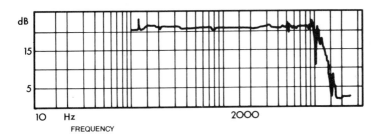

FIG. 11-6.   Frequency response of 6-inch speaker with compressor control.

input to the speaker in the direction of obtaining a constant speaker output to the microphone under test. The result, illustrated in Fig. 11-6, is an output varying around some small value, with the variation in output dependent on the sensitivity of the compressor input of the oscillator. (Audiologists will recognize the system just described as the same one used in evaluating hearing aids.)

As stated previously, there is no standard method of specifying frequency response, but usually the range is specified by the two frequency limits within which the output varies by no more than some specified amount of amplitude: for example, "20 to 20,000 Hz ± 3 dB." This can be translated as a frequency response which varies within + 3 dB and − 3 dB, and no more, between the frequencies of 20 Hz and 20,000 Hz (this would be an excellent microphone).

In most clinical situations a microphone that is relatively flat from 100 Hz to 8,000 Hz is adequate, although it may happen that a sharp /s/ might be lost unless the range is slightly above this. It is the subjective impression of some people that a microphone will produce better recordings if its response extends to 12,000–15,000 Hz. Fig. 8-2 (see p. 137) shows the frequency response for a very good, and very expensive, condensor microphone. If one accepts the − 15 dB line as an arbitrary reference, then this microphone varies 0 dB at approximately 30 Hz, + 3 dB at 15,000 Hz, and −3 dB again at about 25,000 Hz, so its response is ±3 dB from 30 to 25,000 Hz. The sensitivity of 0 dB means that when a sound pressure of 1 dyne/cm² is present at the face of the microphone, then the microphone output is 1 V. If it is less, the decibel value is computed and it is given as minus so many decibels. Most microphones have sensitivities of − 50 to − 60 dB.

DIRECTIONAL CHARACTERISTICS

The directional characteristic of a microphone is a measure of the relative response of the microphone to sound from various locations around it. It is measured by placing the microphone in front of a speaker and plotting the microphone's voltage output as the speaker is rotated around the microphone at a constant distance. This procedure is usually automated, just as is the procedure for measuring frequency response. A level recorder with polar paper is used, and the paper drive motor is coupled to a motor that either rotates the microphone on an axis or moves the speaker around the microphone. *Polar paper* is graph paper on which a series of concentric circles represents the axis specifying the sound pressure. The other axis of the graph is the angle from which the sound is generated with respect to the position of the microphone. Usually a line drawn from the center of the circles to the top of the paper is considered 0°. A point along this line then would represent the sound pressure of a sound from a speaker directly in front of the microphone. If the speaker were behind the microphone, the output would be plotted along a line from the center of the circles to the bottom of the paper. Thus, as the output is plotted, the speaker is moving in step with the azimuth values on the chart. The result is a polar response curve as shown in Fig. 11-7.

To read this graph, choose a value of frequency, which is the parameter noted at the right, and follow the line around the microphone. For ex-

FIG. 11-7.   Directional characteristics of a microphone. (Courtesy Bruel & Kjaer Instruments, Inc., Marlborough, Mass.)

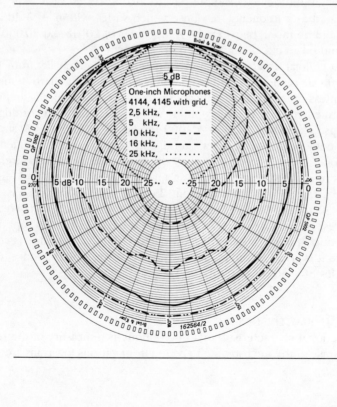

ample, at 5 kHz the response of the microphone at 0° is 75 dB sound pressure level (SPL). At 180°, at the bottom of the graph, the response is approximately 3 dB less or 72 dB. At 25 kHz the response at 0° is 75 dB, but the response drops to 58 dB at 300° and to 0 dB at the back of the microphone (180°).

Some microphones, described below, are designed to have certain directional characteristics.

Omnidirectional Microphones

These microphones are sensitive to sound from any angle around them. There may often be bumps and valleys in their polar response curves, but nothing very discrepant.

Cardioid Microphones

Cardioid microphones are so named because their polar response curves are heart-shaped. These microphones will pick up sound from in front of them but little from behind them; thus they can be used in public address systems because they are sensitive to the speaker but not to the noises of the crowd on the other side of the footlights.

Super Directional Microphones

So-called shotgun microphones and those microphones with parabolic reflectors similar to radar dishes are extremely directional and sensitive. They are specialized microphones, however, and are seldom encountered.

Techniques for Evaluating Loudspeakers

FREQUENCY RESPONSE

The same characteristics that are measured in input transducers are measured in output transducers. The first characteristic is frequency response. This is measured by placing a microphone, whose characteristics are specified, in front of the speaker. The speaker is then fed varying frequencies, and the output at each of these frequencies is measured. Usually this procedure is automated just as in the microphone measurement procedure. When evaluating microphones, a constant amplitude output from the speaker is desired. In like manner, when evaluating speakers, a flat frequency response in the calibration microphone is desired. The oscillator is driven by a motor that also moves the chart paper. The output of the speaker is received by a microphone that drives a pen recorder. The result is a frequency response plot, which is the frequency sensitivity of the speaker and microphone. If the microphone is chosen for a flat frequency response, any amplitude variation that appears results from the speaker.

EFFICIENCY

One characteristic of speakers to be considered is efficiency. A loud-speaker (plus its enclosure) is a device with reactance as well as resistance to energy flow. Its frequency response must be compensated if its output is not to be distorted. Sometimes this is accomplished by "tuning" the enclosure—that is, by having its frequency response complement that of the speaker itself so that the joint response is closer to flat. Otherwise, the enclosure is designed to provide high resistance to the operation of the speaker. A highly resistive enclosure minimizes the influence of the speaker's reactance(s) so that the frequency response is more nearly flat; the speaker plus enclosure are very inefficient, however, necessitating a great deal of power to produce adequate sound. Whereas it might require 2 or 3 W of power to fill a living room with sound from an efficient speaker, a highly inefficient one (such as many of the small, high-fidelity, "bookshelf" speakers) may require 40 or 50 W of power. Most of that energy is used in overcoming the speaker's resistance and serves to fill the room with heat rather than music. The measure of efficiency can be taken for one or more loudspeakers by setting the output level of the speaker to some predetermined level, typically done in an anechoic chamber, and then measuring the power input required by the speaker to achieve that output.

A common method for specifying loudspeakers is to apply a sine wave signal so that the speaker is delivering its maximum output level, as specified by the designer, and measuring the sound pressure level. The resultant value is used as the *SPL-at-rated-output* specification. Another method is to apply 1 W to the speaker and use the resultant SPL as an indicator of output efficiency. This latter method is uncommon today.

HARMONIC DISTORTION

Harmonic distortion of loudspeakers is another assessment of interest and is measured as in amplifier evaluation. Again, a very good measurement microphone must be used to prevent contamination of the acoustic signal.

DYNAMIC RANGE

An additional characteristic of occasional use in evaluating a loudspeaker is its dynamic range. Once the speaker reproduces a signal loud enough to be heard, how much more intensely can the signal be reproduced without measurably increasing the distortion of the output? This value is usually expressed as so many decibels at 1% or 0.1% distortion.

TRANSIENT RESPONSE

Yet another measure of speaker quality, particularly important for research in speech and hearing science, is the transducer's transient response—its ability to reproduce signals with high frequency content. A moment's reflection reminds us that high frequency sinusoids are more rapidly changing signals than lower frequency waves. In like manner, the ability of any transducer to follow a rapidly changing transient event— such as an electrical impulse or a voiceless plosive—is related to its frequency response and to its dynamic range as well. There is no standard for measurement of transient distortion, and several different procedures have appeared in studies in the literature.

DIRECTIONAL CHARACTERISTICS

The directional characteristics of loudspeakers are especially critical because of the interaction of frequency response measurement and directivity. That is, if the frequency response is assessed at one point in front of the speaker it is important to know how much this response will change at other points. Loudspeakers often have a tendency to exhibit peculiar narrow spatial patterns of increased or decreased projection.

The directivity of a speaker is measured just as with microphones, but the measurement microphone is moved around the speaker. A polar response chart as shown in Fig. 11-8 will be obtained. Note that the response at high frequencies shows narrow lanes of increased energy. This peculiarity is called *beaming* and, of course, should be avoided because

FIG. 11-8.   Typical directional characteristics of a loudspeaker. (Courtesy Bruel & Kjaer Instruments, Inc., Marlborough, Mass.)

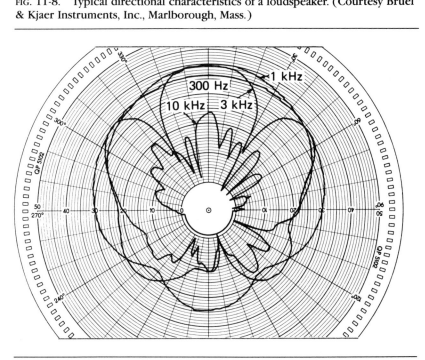

if the listener is even slightly off the 0° axis, the output can drop by 20 dB.

Suggested Reading

Beranek, L. L.   *Acoustic Measurements.* New York: Wiley, 1962.

Crowhurst, N. H.   *Audio Measurements.* New York: Gernsback, 1958.

Hassall, J. R., and Zaveri, K.   *Acoustic Noise Measurements.* Copenhagen: Bruel & Kjaer, 1979.

Langford-Smith, F.   *Radiotron Designer's Handbook.* Harrison, N.J.: RCA, 1953.

Malmstadt, H. V., and Enke, C. G.   *Electronics for Scientists.* New York: Benjamin, 1963.

Malmstadt, H. V., and Enke, C. G.   *Digital Electronics for Scientists.* New York: Benjamin, 1969.

Peterson, A. P. G.   *Handbook of Noise Measurement.* Concord, Mass.: Genrad, 1980.

Randall, R. B   *Frequency Analysis.* Copenhagen: Bruel & Kjaer, 1979.

V. Common Laboratory Instruments

12. Laboratory Equipment

Electrophysiologic Recorders

One application of amplifier technology commonly found in the speech and hearing science laboratory is the electrophysiologic recorder. This recorder comprises an impressive array of equipment but is conceptually quite simple.

GENERAL INSTRUMENTATION

The front end of the electrophysiologic recorder is composed of a set of couplers into which electrodes connect to pick up the electrical activity associated with neural transmission, as in electroencephalography, or with muscle movement, as in electromyography or electrocardiography, or couplers that accommodate various transducers to change mechanical or aerodynamic signals into electrical signals, as in measurement of air pressure or blood flow. The electrical signals must then be amplified and analyzed, measured, or stored. Fig. 12-1 is a picture of one type of electrophysiologic recording system. It can be broken down into four basic parts. First, the *couplers* are devices that match the impedances and other necessary electrical characteristics to the preamplifiers. The couplers are shown at the top left of Fig. 12-1 with cables leading to them. The second part of the system, the *preamplifiers,* is necessary because many of the signals to be recorded are extremely weak, sometimes only 2 to 4 μV. The preamplifiers boost the signals, feed them to the power amplifiers, and are visible in Fig. 12-1 as six knobs in a row just below the couplers. The third part, the *power amplifiers* just mentioned, are located below the preamplifiers and provide enough power to drive the fourth part, the *galvanometers.* Galvanometers are similar to meter

193

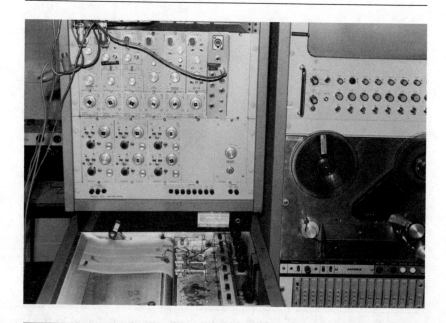

FIG. 12-1.   A six-channel electrophysiologic recorder (left) and large-screen oscilloscope (upper right) with seven-channel FM tape recorder (lower right).

movements (see Chap.7), but they have small capillary pens instead of a needle. These pens are poised above a paper chart, which is part of a roll of paper and is moved by a *paper drive*. This consists of a motor and various gears so that the paper may be moved at a variety of speeds in order to capture the pattern drawn by the pen.

Fig. 12-2 is a block diagram of the system. Note that this system has four essentially similar channels. Some recorders have as many as twelve channels or as few as one. In the speech laboratory it is usually desirable to have at least two, and preferably four, channels. As the examples in Chapter 16 will clarify, we usually monitor several sets of muscles when performing electromyographic measurements, and to record simultaneously, for example, four sets of muscles requires that many inputs. In addition, during assessment of air flow and pressure, the measures of choice are most often intraoral air pressure, nasal airflow, and oral airflow. Thus the desirability of multiple inputs should be obvious.

The couplers appear as in Fig. 12-3. Note that there are sensitivity adjustments available and low- and highpass filtering. These controls are especially important in electroencephalographic recording to eliminate the stray fields that interfere with the extremely small voltages present in the electroencephalogram (EEG).

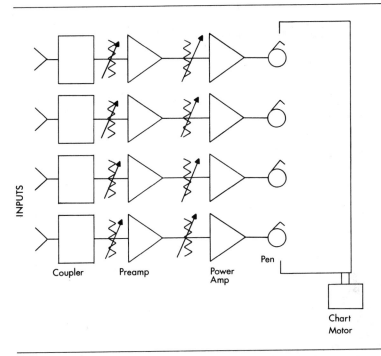

INPUTS

Coupler   Preamp   Power   Pen
                                    Amp

Chart
Motor

FIG. 12-2.   Block diagram of four-channel electrophysiologic recorder.

The preamplifiers and power amplifiers both have gain controls and possibly might have additional filters. The units of an electrophysiologic recording system typically plug into a rack as in Fig. 12-1; all the interconnections are made within the cabinet. This eliminates the tangle of cords that would result otherwise. The power amplifier has provisions for feeding a signal directly into it, bypassing the preamplifier.

ELECTRODES

Many of the parameters of speech that are of interest to clinicians are related to electrical signals within the organism. The electromyogram (EMG) is correlated with muscular activity and can serve as an excellent indicator of the strength of muscular contraction. The EEG arises from electrical activity in the brain; therefore, if taken during stimulation of the senses, the EEG, by generalization, can indicate sensory input necessary for perception. In order to examine these electrical signals, they must be coupled from the organism to the equipment that amplifies and displays them.

Electrodes are used to route the electrical activity from a portion of the body to a wire carrying the signal to an amplifier. Although this may seem to be a simple task, the problems involved can be many. First, there

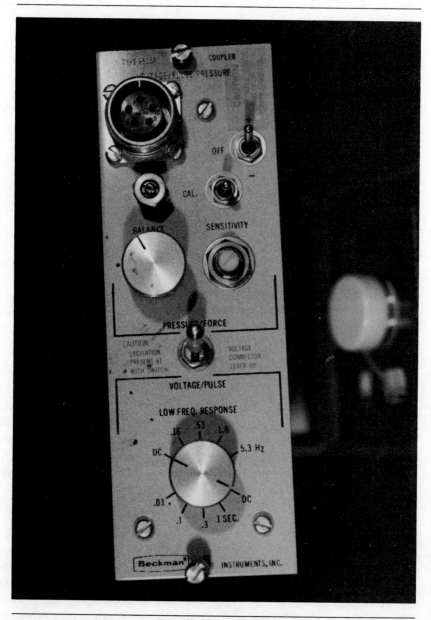

FIG. 12-3.   An all-purpose coupler used in the six-channel recorder of Fig. 12-1.

is the problem of isolating the area to be measured. The body is full of electrical activity, each muscle having an electrical signal associated with it; the end organs associated with the sensory inputs all generate an electrical signal. Thus, placing an electrode on the scalp and measuring the signal present provides only an indication of the electrical activity at this location; it does not ensure that the signal did not originate at quite a distance from the position at which the electrode was applied. The heart muscle, for example, generates an extremely strong electrical signal and often contaminates signals from electrodes placed in locations as distant as the ends of the fingers.

In some laboratories *intracellular electrodes* are used. These consist of needles inserted under the skin or into the organ being measured. The intracellular electrode does provide a better coupling of the electrical signal than does the surface electrode, but there are risks associated with inserting needles into a subject. Also, some organs (e.g., heart and eye) cannot be assessed with this technique for obvious reasons.

Another problem associated with electrodes is *voltaic action*. This is best explained by reference to an experiment that is sometimes carried out in elementary physics classes. A silver coin is placed on a copper coin. The two dissimilar metals in combination with body acids form a small battery that can be seen as a DC voltage. The DC voltage will appear at the input of the amplifier as an offset and also will cause the pens of the galvanometer to be deflected. This may shift the operating range of the amplifier and generate severe distortion and artifacts. So in general, speech researchers use silver electrodes or silver with a chloride plating. In some cases, gold electrodes are much better, but this is not the case for EEG and EMG recording.

The *disk electrode* usually has the shape shown in Fig. 12-4. It has a concave shape and a paste is smeared into the depression. The paste, called *electrode paste,* matches the chemical composition of the skin surface to the electrode. Some electrode paste is adhesive so that the electrode will stick in place. When using nonadhesive paste, circular adhesive patches are placed over the electrode and stuck to the skin. (It is good practice to also place adhesive tape on the electrode wire so that it will not flex and pull the electrode loose.)

The disk electrode is adequate for most EEG or galvanic skin resistance (GSR) measurements, but, for assessing muscle activity, another type of electrode has become popular recently. This electrode consists of a paint that is applied to the surface of the skin. A fine wire is then inserted into the paint. When the paint dries, the wire is held in place. The wire is then attached to the amplifier. The paint consists of equal parts of silver powder, Duco cement, and acetone. This is a very useful type of electrode as it adds very little mass to the surface on which it is applied. It does suffer from the same problems that all surface electrodes have when trying to couple EMG signals: it is difficult to determine what muscle

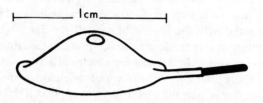

FIG. 12-4.   A typical disk electrode.

potential is actually being coupled because in most areas of the speech musculature there are many layers from many different muscles lying in close proximity or even over one another. For this reason, most speech scientists will use intracellular electrodes in assessing EMGs.

Pneumotachographs

Occasionally, the clinician must assess airflow, either in normal or non-normal speakers. Only a small amount of air moves during phonation, so that its measurement requires a sensitive measurement system. The device typically used in the measurement task is called a *pneumotachograph* and consists of a face mask with an acoustic resistance (an acoustic resistance, like an electrical resistance, offers constant opposition to the flow of air through it, regardless of the frequency, and results in a drop in air pressure through it). The acoustic resistance is connected to a tube from the mask. A transducer that turns difference in air pressure into electrical pressure (i.e., voltage) monitors the pressure change across the resistance and gives an indication of the amount of air across the resistance by displaying the pressure drop. In the pneumotachograph, pressure can be applied to both sides of the diaphragm, whereas in the more common pressure transducers, such as microphones, the rear of the diaphragm is sealed. With the differential transducer of the pneumotachograph, there will be no output so long as the pressure is equal on the two sides of the diaphragm, no matter how great or small the total pressure may be. When air flows through the resistance (R), however, a pressure change (E) will occur. By Ohm's law, airflow (I) = E/R.

Fig. 12-5 illustrates this arrangement. The mask is worn by the person who is talking, and the output of the mask passes through R. The tubes connect the pressure transducer (T) across the resistance, and the electrical output of the transducer, which is equivalent to the pressure change across R, is fed into an amplifier (A) and then to a recording device, usually a strip-chart recorder. The unit is calibrated by passing a known rate of airflow through the resistance and noting the deflection

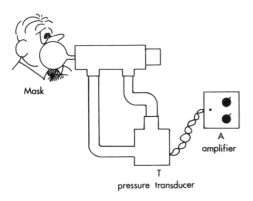

Mask

A
amplifier

T
pressure transducer

FIG. 12-5.   General arrangement for airflow measurement.

on the chart. It is assumed that the pen deflections will be linear, so that one-half the deflection is one-half the airflow rate. If the parameter of interest is the total amount of air (equivalent to energy), the amplifier output is fed to an integrator, a device that stores the charge, and the result is the sum of the flow rate times the duration of the signal. In this case, a capacitor connected to the electrical output of the amplifier stores the charge, which can then be measured and recorded.

The pneumotachograph is used in conjunction with a standard electrophysiologic recorder. That is, it is connected to a high-gain amplifier that also provides a polarizing voltage necessary for the pressure transducer and a voltage to heat the acoustic resistance. The heating prevents drift in the measure due to the cooling effects of air passing through the transducer. Usually, a heater is unnecessary as only a small quantity of air flows.

Ultrasonics

Speech research is often concerned with the size, shape, and volume of a cavity that cannot be viewed from the outside. For example, it is not possible to optically examine the approximation of the vocal folds and the shape of the immediately superior portions of the laryngeal cavity without the confounding instrumentation necessary for indirect laryngoscopy. In cases such as these, ultrasonics are useful.

An *ultrasonic system* is similar to sonar and radar in that an echo is used as the indicator of a signal. Ultrasonic equipment consists of a device that houses both an output and an input transducer. A burst of high-frequency energy is emitted from the output transducers and begins traversing the body over which it has been placed. When high-frequency

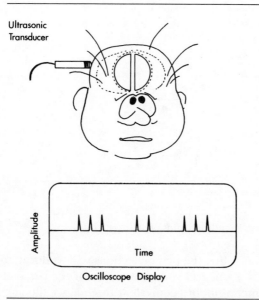

FIG. 12-6. Ultrasonic scanning of the cranium and resulting display.

waves pass from the boundary of one material to another, some of the energy is reflected from the boundary as the wave enters. This reflection, or echo, occurs at each interface; an interface is the boundary between two materials. Fig. 12-6 shows an ultrasonic signal passing through the cranial cavity. There is an echo at each interface: the skin, the skull bone, the surface of the brain, the other side of the brain, the skull bone and finally the skin on the side opposite the transducer. If the echoes are plotted on an oscilloscope so that the travel time of the pulse is preserved, an indication of the distance the pulse had to travel through each material will be computed, denoting the thickness of each of the materials and the diameter of the brain.

There are some situations in which ultrasonics might not be useful. One is in scanning a cavity that is filled with air. The air interface is about 99% reflective, which means that the pulse will be almost entirely reflected when it hits the boundary between tissue and air cavity. Thus, there is no energy to pass on to give some indications of the size of the cavity. For this reason it is difficult to use an ultrasonic system in scanning the oral cavity or even the largyngeal cavity when the glottis is open. Almost all the detail in the cavity will be lost.

In some cases these pulses, due to the echoes, are converted into spots of light, the intensity of the spot being proportional to the amplitude of the echo. If these are displayed on a scope it is called *Z-axis modulation.* (The Z-axis on an oscilloscope is considered the brightness of the display.) If the scope is adjusted so that only spots due to echoes are pres-

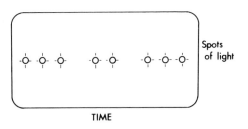

FIG. 12-7. Z-axis modulated display.

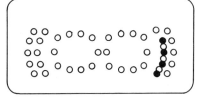

FIG. 12-8. Scanning with z-axis modulation display.

ent, the display appears as in Fig. 12-7. Here the spots of light visible are those at the interfaces of the various media. The separation between the spots is indicative of the thickness of material through which the pulse passes or the size of the cavity.

If now the transducer is slowly moved in a vertical plane and the Z-axis modulation continued, a display such as Fig. 12-8 results. Now an outline of the structures is visible.

Photocells

A useful device in the speech and hearing science laboratory is the *photocell*. This is a unit that serves as a resistance, but the resistance value is a function of the light falling on the cell. If the cell is in the dark, it will have a very high resistance; once it is illuminated the resistance drops appreciably. One use of the photocell is in measuring blood flow. The photocell is placed on one side of a finger and a small lamp is placed on the other side. The light passes through the finger and illuminates the cell. If the cell is connected as in Fig. 12-9, a current will flow, the value of which is determined by the resistance of the photocell. When a large pulse of blood passes through the finger, the cell becomes somewhat darker and the current drops because the resistance of the photocell

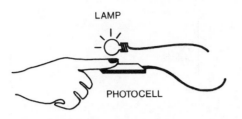

LAMP

PHOTOCELL

FIG. 12-9.   Pulse counter input using photocell.

increases. When the pulse of blood passes, the current increases again, so that there is a decrease in current every time a pulse of blood passes through the finger. The readout that might be plotted on a chart recorder is a series of peaks and valleys associated with the pulse rate.

The photocell is also used on tape recorders (as illustrated in Fig. 12-10) so that the unit stops when there is no more tape on the machine. As long as there is tape between the light and the photocell, the relay is not energized because the resistance is so high that insufficient current can flow. When the tape is no longer present, the relay is energized and breaks the circuit in the play mode, and the machine stops.

The photocell is also used in a technique for determining glottal opening called *transilluminance*. This technique consists of placing a light source against the throat below the thyroid cartilage. (The light source consists of a light shining through a container of water so that the lamp housing in contact with the skin is cool. A strong light source without this safeguard could easily burn the skin.) A photocell attached to a thin cable is placed at the back of the oral cavity above the glottis. If the glottis is open, the light shining through the tissue illuminates the cell and causes the resistance to drop. The cell is connected so that as the glottis opens and closes the cell resistance varies, and the current also varies as a function of the size of the opening. Fig. 12-11 illustrates the technique of transilluminance. As the photocell changes resistance, more or less voltage from the cell's battery appears at the amplifier input.

Laryngographs

The laryngograph is used in a much simpler method than transilluminance for measuring the size of the glottis. This instrument measures the resistance between the two vocal folds and displays the pattern over time on an oscilloscope. Electrodes are placed on either side of the thyroid notch and held in place with a Velcro strap. The electrodes are connected to a processor, which feeds a very small voltage to the electrodes.

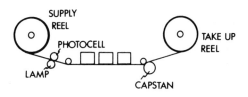

FIG. 12-10. End-of-tape switch using photocell.

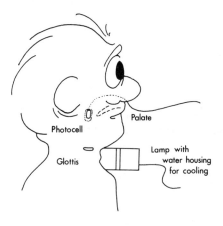

FIG. 12-11. Transilluminance technique for determining glottal opening.

The amount of current that can flow between the two electrodes will be a function of the resistance between them, and this resistance will vary from a very small amount when the vocal folds are touching to a large amount when the folds are far apart. The varying current due to changes in separation of the vocal folds is changed into a varying voltage in the processor, and the output of the processor is then connected to an oscilloscope. The pattern on the oscilloscope will be a beam that will deflect up as the folds move farther apart and down as they move together. With this technique it is possible to obtain a real-time picture of the glottal functioning. The pattern may then be photographed or fed to a computer for further analysis.

Suggested Reading

Borden, G. J., and Harris, K. S. *Speech Science Primer.* Baltimore: Williams & Wilkins, 1984.

Geddes, L. A., and Baker, L. E.   *Bio-medical Instrumentation.* New York: Wiley, 1968.

Lass, N. J. (Ed.).   *Contemporary Issues in Experimental Phonetics.* New York: Academic, 1976.

Lehiste, I. (Ed.).   *Readings in Acoustic Phonetics.* Cambridge, Mass.: MIT Press, 1969.

Lieberman, P.   *Speech Physiology and Acoustic Phonetics: An Introduction.* New York: Macmillan, 1977.

Luchsinger, R., and Arnold, G. E.   *Voice-Speech-Language.* Belmont, Calif.: Wadsworth, 1965.

Mackay, R. S.   *Biomedical Telemetry.* New York: Wiley, 1970.

Minifie, F. D., Hixon, T. J., and Williams, F.   *Normal Aspects of Speech, Hearing and Language.* Englewood Cliffs, N.J.: Prentice-Hall, 1978.

Perkell, J. S.   *Physiology of Speech Production.* Cambridge, Mass.: MIT Press, 1969.

Peterson, H. A., and Marquardt, T. P.   *Appraisal and Diagnosis of Speech and Language Disorders.* Englewood Cliffs, N.J.: Prentice-Hall, 1981.

Venables, P. H., and Martin, I.   *Manual of Psychophysiological Methods.* New York: Elsevier, 1967.

Watkins, K. L., and Zagzebski, J. A.   On-line ultrasonic technique for monitoring tongue movement. *J. Acoust. Soc. Am.* 54:544–547, 1973.

13. The Sound Spectrograph

Three dimensions—change in frequency and amplitude over time—are necessary to specify acoustic signals. Therefore, to assess these dimensions simultaneously in speech or other signals, a three-dimensional display is necessary. Several devices have been created in the last few years that allow for simultaneous display of all three dimensions, but the oldest device still in use, and the most common, is the sound spectrograph. Although several different units are available, the unit we describe is the Kay Sound Sonagraph, which is manufactured by the Kay Elemetrics Corporation (Pine Brook, N. J.).

The Sonagraph

Consider first an overview of the system. A sound spectrograph requires the following components:

1. A recorder to store and sample repeatedly the signal being analyzed
2. A filter to analyze the signal's frequency content
3. Metering circuitry to measure the signal amplitude at each frequency, or in each frequency band, for each time interval sampled
4. A visual display device to present simultaneously all three dimensions

OPERATING PRINCIPLES

The sound spectrograph works by incorporating a series of clever design features. First, it records a signal in a magnetic medium along an edge of a rotating turntable. The same rotating turntable also has a drum on it that holds the display paper so that the position of the portion of the signal being reproduced remains precisely related to the position of the display of that portion of the signal (the importance of this linkage will become apparent).

Second, the spectrograph uses only one filter, instead of a series of filters, to analyze the entire frequency content of the signal. The sophistication of the device is revealed by the fact that the filter does not vary in center frequency in order to move gradually through the frequency range it must analyze; rather, the filter has a fixed frequency, and the signal frequency range is gradually shifted through it as will be explained shortly. The importance of this filter is that it has precisely the desired characteristics. A movable filter would involve making compromises, and a series of equally good filters would be too costly.

Finally, concentric with the turntable on which the signal is being recorded is a shaft that performs two functions. First, it changes the operating system so that the frequency analysis gradually shifts from low frequencies to higher frequencies as the turntable rotates. Second, the shaft moves a marking stylus to different locations on the recording paper as a function of the frequency being examined. Thus, lower frequencies will be recorded at the bottom of the paper and higher frequencies at the top.

To begin, a microphone feeds the signal to the tape-recording circuitry, and the signal is recorded on a magnetic medium bonded to the edge of a turntable with a 2.4-second rotation period during recording. Therefore, only 2.4 seconds of speech can be recorded at a time. Newer models of the Kay Sound Sonagraph allow the operator to place a longer tape recording on a peripheral tape recorder and record and analyze the signal in 2.4-second segments until the entire tape is analyzed.

After the signal is recorded on the edge of the disk, the operator switches to the reproduce mode, which connects a playback head into the circuit. The signal is taken from the disk with a reproduction speed twelve times faster than the recording rotation rate and fed into the processor.

Once the signal is recorded, the drum speed is accelerated so that the recorded signal frequencies are increased by a factor of twelve. The signal frequencies are then fed to a device called a *balanced modulator,* in which they are combined with a variable frequency from 200 to 296 kHz generated by the Sonagraph. The output of the modulator is a combination of the sums and differences of the recorded signal and the internal oscillator. This combination signal is then fed into a very sharp filter called an *intermediate frequency* (IF) *filter.*

To clarify the next step let us use some specific numbers as an example. Consider that the input signal that is recorded contains frequencies of 100, 500, and 900 Hz. When speeded up during analysis, these frequencies become 1,200, 6,000, and 10,800 Hz, respectively. If the internal oscillator is generating a frequency of 200 kHz, the sums of the recorded frequencies added to the internal oscillator frequency by the balanced modulator become 201,200, 206,000, and 210,800 Hz, and the differences become 198,800, 194,000, and 189,200 Hz, respectively. Now consider that the IF filter is tuned to 200 kHz. If the filter sees some energy at that frequency, it will allow it to pass to an amplifier that is connected to a stylus. The amplifier supplies a very large voltage to the stylus, and a spark will jump if the stylus is placed near the ground side of the circuit. The ground side of the circuit is the drum on the machine, and a piece of heat-sensitive paper is interposed between the stylus and the drum. The spark jumps and burns the paper. If there is a great deal of energy passing through the filter, the spark will be large and the burn very black. If there is only a small amount of energy, the spark will be weak and will only slightly burn the paper. Thus, the relative intensity of the signal is displayed by the darkness of the burn. Now, as the drum turns, the internal oscillator is tuned because a resistance is connected to a screw drive that is driven by the same motor moving the drum. The internal oscillator is tuned to a higher frequency as the drum rotates, and the sums and differences will constantly change. If the internal oscillator is now tuned to 201,200 Hz, the difference frequencies are 200,000, 195,200, and 190,400 Hz. The IF filter sees energy at its 200,000 Hz tuning, so a burn takes place. As the drum rotates the internal oscillator eventually reaches a frequency of 202,000 Hz. The differences now become 200,800, 196,000, and 191,200 Hz. Once again the IF filter sees no energy, so no signal is passed to burn the paper. So that the frequency dimension is maintained on the vertical axis, the same carriage that moves the tuning resistor also moves the stylus on the paper, and, as the frequency increases, the stylus moves up the paper. (It should be noted that there is a switch on the Sonagraph that allows the frequency to be inverted so that as the stylus moves up the paper, the frequency being burned goes down.) These figures, in conjunction with this lengthy description, should have made clear a rather simple, but clever, analyzing technique.

There are many variations in the basic operation of the Sonagraph. A few will be described below.

FILTERS

Probably the most frequently used option on the sound spectrograph is that of a change in filter bandwidth. The internal circuitry of the spectrograph allows two choices in the width of the filter: the standard bandwidth of 300 Hz and one that is 45 Hz.

The nature of the speech wave causes it to be portrayed very differently when a narrow filter, rather than a broad filter, is used. As we know, the typical speech wave is composed of a fundamental frequency and a large number of harmonically related overtones (or partials). The fundamental frequency of the habitual pitch of the typical male voice, for example, is likely to be approximately 130 Hz, and the lower frequency components of the partial series above the fundamental would, then, be 260, 390, 520, 650, 780, and 910 Hz, and so on. Further, fundamental vocal frequency variations (called *jitter*) in the male voice are typically 7 to 10 Hz, so the fundamental frequency would, if the voice were sustained, vary from approximately 125 to 135 Hz, and the partials would then "wobble" from 250 to 270, 375 to 405, 500 to 540, 625 to 675, 750 to 810, and 875 to 945 Hz, and so on.

The narrow filter is narrower than the separation between partials, but the broad filter is not. When the broad filter is used, the energy from more than a single partial falls into the passband region of the filter at any time, and the graphed output is a broad band of energies, as shown in Fig. 13-1. Using the narrow filter, however, results in only a single partial being in the passband at any moment in time so that the graph portrays individual partials of the vocal output. (See Fig. 13-3, where the bottom of the graph depicts the same recorded signal as shown in Fig. 13-1 but where the narrow filter setting is in use.)

SECTIONER

The sectioner is a circuit that allows the operator to examine one or several particular points in time of the recorded signal and to produce a histogram of the amplitude of the various frequencies at that instant or those instants. The histogram is produced by adjusting magnets on the top of the drum at the point or points of interest. When the drum rotates in the reproduction mode, each time the magnet passes a small switch placed near the rotating drum a circuit is closed and the energy present at the output of the filter at that instant is sampled. The stylus serves as the route to discharge the energy and burns the paper for a duration proportional to the amplitude. The result is a graph similar to the one shown in Fig. 13.2. Note that the vertical dimension is frequency and that the amplitude is now equivalent to the length of the line burned. Time is no longer assessed. It is possible to sample several points on the recording with the sectioner, but the recordings cannot be too close together or they will overlap and obscure one another. A section is a useful display for determining the center of bell-shaped bands that might otherwise appear as black smears on the normal display.

AMPLITUDE DISPLAY

The amplitude display is one in which the overall amplitude of the signal at each moment in time is drawn on the paper immediately above the normal pattern without regard for its frequency content. This display is particularly useful for examining stress patterns. To obtain the display, the filter is removed from the circuit and is replaced by a comparator circuit, which operates in the following manner: as the drum revolves and the stylus gradually but progressively ascends, each height of the

209

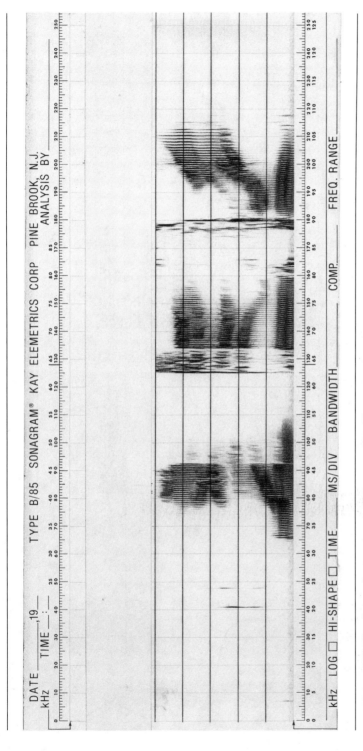

FIG. 13-1. Wide-band speech spectrogram. (Courtesy Kay Elemetrics Corp., Pine Brook, N.J.)

210

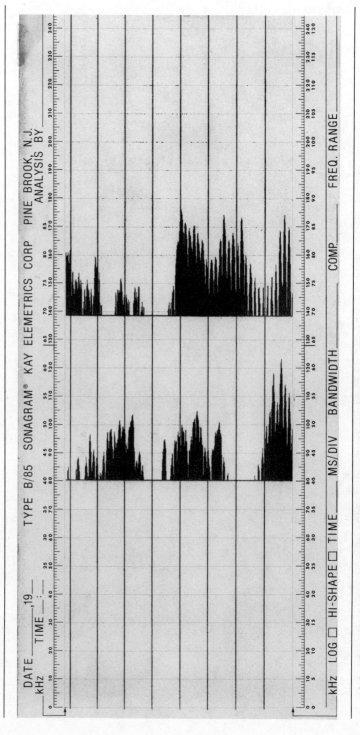

FIG. 13-2. Sectioned display of a speech spectrogram. (Courtesy Kay Elemetrics Corp., Pine Brook, N.J.)

stylus is made to represent some magnitude of signal energy. The amount of energy in the signal is compared with the magnitude of energy represented by the stylus height, and, if the energies are equal, the stylus momentarily receives marking voltage and burns a mark on the paper. If the energy of the signal is either more or less than the required amount for that stylus height, no marking voltage is delivered to the stylus. As the drum turns and the stylus ascends, a mark is made at each location where vocalization is present, at a height determined by the signal energy. When the final pattern is examined, however, the result is a contour like that at the top of Fig. 13-3.

AGNELLOGRAPH

Another display is called the agnellograph and consists of a trace similar to the amplitude display. In this case, however, the amplitude is that from a recording of a pressure signal from a pressure transducer placed in either the oral or nasal cavity, not that from a recording of the acoustic signal. Other than this, the pattern is the same as the amplitude display, and the result is a pattern of pressure changes displayed immediately above the normal three-dimensional display.

CONTOUR DISPLAY

The last variation on the spectrographic pattern is the contour display. This display is desirable because the heat-sensitive paper used with the normal display has only a limited dynamic range. The range of intensity between no-burn and maximum burn of the paper is only 6 dB. The range of speech amplitudes is much greater than this (as much as 35-40 dB), which means that it is often difficult to distinguish whether, in fact, there is an amplitude difference between two dark burns. Therefore, if the spectrograph unit is set so that the small amplitudes present at the output of the filter will burn the paper, the more intense amplitudes will burn too black and thus all the high-amplitude signals will appear the same. Similarly, if the unit is set so that the high-amplitude signals burn so that they may be distinguished, the weaker signals will not burn at all. To overcome some of these problems, the original spectrograph units were equipped with an automatic gain control circuitry, which essentially compressed the dynamic range of speech so that weak signals were made slightly higher in amplitude and the high amplitude signals were attenuated slightly. For routine clinical examinations this does not interfere greatly with analysis, but something that causes less distortion is necessary for precise measurements. The solution arrived at in the sound spectrograph is a unit that displays a pattern very similar to a topographic map. The signal fed to the stylus is adjusted so that only one of seven voltages will be present, dependent on the output of a device that has the total amplitude broken into seven segments, each 6 dB apart. Fig. 13-4 shows how the amplitude is analyzed. If the signal from the filter falls

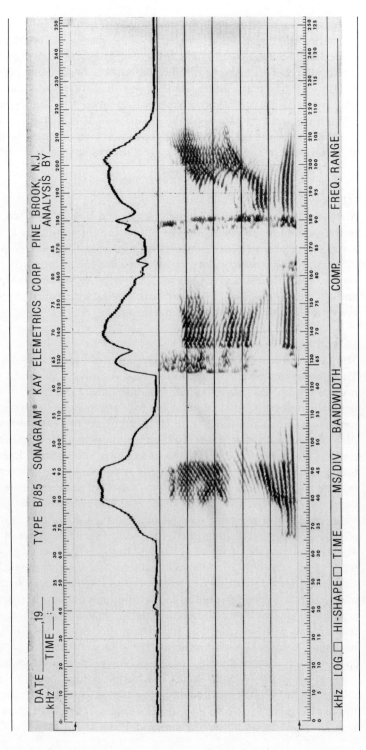

FIG. 13-3. Amplitude display above a narrow-band speech spectrogram. (Courtesy Kay Elemetrics Corp., Pine Brook, N.J.)

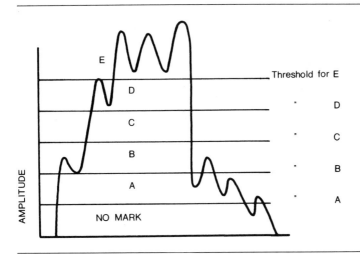

FIG. 13-4. Thresholds for contour.

in area A, the amplitude associated with A is fed to the stylus. The amplitude to the stylus will be the same regardless of where in the area the input signal falls. If the signal is more intense, it may fall into area B. In these cases, a more intense signal will be fed to the stylus. The result is a burn pattern that consists of several degrees of darkness, just as a topographic map shows altitude by various shades of gray or by various colors. To improve the readability of the contour display, the unit also outlines each of the various contours with a dense unbroken, black line. Fig. 13-5 shows a contour display. Notice how much easier it is to read, how much easier it is to determine when the amplitude of a signal has changed, and how clearly defined the formants of the vowels become.

The Digital Spectrograph

Kay Elemetrics has recently developed a digital sound spectrograph that provides many advantages over the Sonagraph, which has been described. One of the principal advantages to digital processing is that digital filters may be used, which center on specific frequencies and can have very precisely defined bandwidths. Also, the skirts of the filter are essentially vertical so the filter either passes a signal or it does not: there is no slope at the upper and lower frequency limits. Another advantage is the ability to locate a specific segment of a recording because the material is stored in a digital buffer that is akin to a file cabinet. Each segment of the recorded sample is assigned two numbers. One number is

214

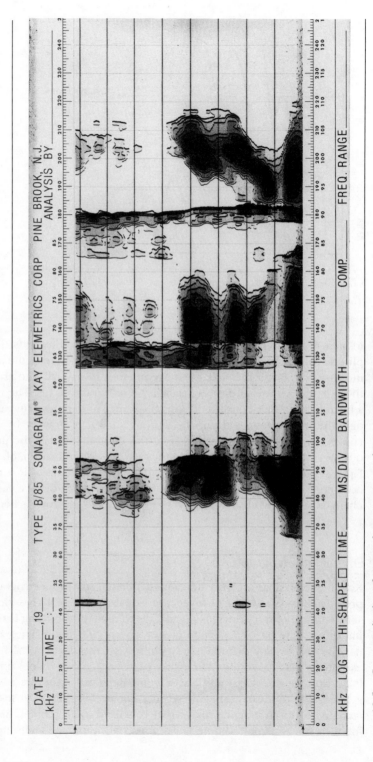

FIG. 13-5. Contour display of a speech spectrogram. (Courtesy Kay Elemetrics Corp., Pine Brook, N.J.)

the value of the amplitude, the other an address where the value is stored. Thus, to locate a segment it is necessary only to enter an address value and the processor will find the value at that address. To locate a syllable, a series of addresses is entered, and the machine locates the series and moves it to another area for reproduction. A further advantage of the digital buffer is that segments may be moved around. That is, a syllable from one place may be combined with a syllable from another. The shuffling has proved highly valuable in research on human linguistic and phonetic processing. The digital machine is also faster than the mechanical system previously used because it changes analysis parameters digitally. The limiting factor in analysis speed is the change of parameters, so the new machine can present an adequate display in about one-fifth of the time needed by the older machine.

Real-Time Spectrum Analyzers

Real-time spectrum analyzers are a new breed of analyzers that has become available in the last few years. These machines allow the spectrum of a signal to be examined as the signal is produced by passing the signal through a series of continuous narrow-band filters and displaying the outputs of these filters on an oscilloscope screen. Fig. 13-6 shows a current version of the real-time analyzer. The various controls below the screen allow the operator to select which frequencies will be displayed on the screen, the time alloted to the displays, and various other parameters of the signal processing. The version shown here allows display of the waveform, too.

There are essentially two types of real-time analyzers. The earlier real-time spectrum analyzers contain a bank of narrow-band (usually one-third octave) filters. The outputs of these filters are then fed to a device called a *multiplexer*. The multiplexer switches each of the filter outputs, in turn, to the screen at a particular location so that the result is a spectrum. The multiplexer operates at a high speed so that the pattern on the screen appears to be stable.

The latest real-time analyzers operate by converting the signal to a digital signal and then performing the filtering operations digitally. The result is much finer frequency discrimination, selectable filter bandwidths and center frequencies, and filters with very sharp skirts. Their major advantage is that the parameters of the machine can all be changed by switches, so that an infinite range of signals may be examined. The only limitation of this type of processing is the rate at which the input signal is converted into a digital signal. Mathematical analyses specify that the sampling rate must be at least twice that of the highest frequency in the signal. Thus, for a 15-kHz signal, the digitizer must operate at 30 kHz. A rate of 30 kHz is not difficult to obtain, but there may be problems at

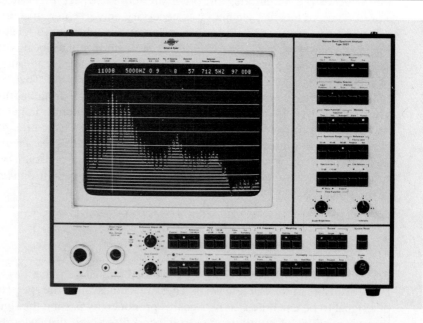

FIG. 13-6.   A real-time spectrum analyzer. (Courtesy Bruel & Kjaer Instruments, Inc., Marlborough, Mass.)

higher rates, so other systems may be used. Fortunately, for our analyses, 30 kHz is fine.

Suggested Reading

Flanagan, J. L.   *Speech Analysis, Synthesis and Perception.* New York: Springer-Verlag, 1965.

Ladafoged, P.   *Elements of Acoustic Phonetics.* Chicago: University of Chicago Press, 1962.

Lehiste, I. (Ed.).   *Readings in Acoustic Phonetics.* Cambridge, Mass.: MIT Press, 1969.

Potter, R. K., Kopp, G. A., and Green, H.   *Visible Speech.* New York: VanNostrand, 1947.

14. Computers

Computers provide many functions impossible to obtain any other way in the speech and hearing science laboratory. This chapter provides a brief overview of computer operation and application. For more details, the student should refer to the suggested reading list at the end of the chapter. The student might also investigate classes in computer operation and programming. Most universities and technical schools, and some computer manufacturers, offer courses for students who have little engineering background.

There are two general types of computers: *analog* and *digital.* The latter type is the type usually being referred to when computers are spoken of. The analog computer is still useful, though uncommon. It merits some consideration for two reasons. First, study of the analog computer offers a focused way of reinforcing many principles underlying general circuit analysis. Second, one application of the analog computer is in synthesizing speech, so that studying this particular application assists our understanding of speech as well as our understanding of an electrical analog of the vocal tract itself.

Analog Computers

The analog computer performs various mathematical operations on voltages that are analogs of the quantities under consideration. A simple example would be one in which an analog computer determines the sum of 2 plus 2. The operation would consist of adding a voltage of 2 V to another voltage of 2 V and reading the answer on a voltmeter at the

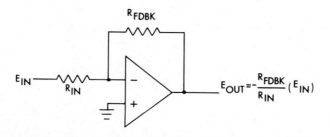

$$E_{OUT} = -\frac{R_{FDBK}}{R_{IN}}(E_{IN})$$

FIG. 14-1.   Block diagram of the basic connections to an operational amplifier. See text for details.

output. To subtract 5 from 9, a voltage of 9 V is fed to an amplifier to be summed with a voltage of 5 that has previously been routed through an amplifier that inverts the value, changing it to −5. When these are summed, the voltmeter would read 4 V.

The heart of the analog computer is the *operational amplifier,* which was discussed earlier in Chapter 4. Recall from Chapter 4 that an operational amplifier contains two input terminals, one positive and one negative. The positive input accepts a voltage, and the amplified output is the same polarity as the input. The negative input results in an amplified output of opposite polarity, an *inverted output.*

The other parts of the analog computer consist of the sources of voltage that provide the values to be computed, the balancing circuits to ensure stability of the amplifiers, and the readout devices. The readout devices are voltmeters, chart recorders, and oscilloscopes.

To perform the first example (2 + 2 V), an amplifier is set up to act as a summer. Several inputs can be connected simultaneously, and the output will equal the sum of the inputs. The amplifier gain can be adjusted by controlling the value of a feedback resistor R_{fdbk} and the value or values of one or more input resistors R_{input}. The gain is determined by the equation, Gain = R_{fdbk}/R_{input}. If the two resistors are equal in value, the gain of the amplifier is 1. Fig. 14-1 shows the arrangement of the amplifier with a gain of 1. Fig. 14-2 shows the amplifier as a summer.

To subtract, a value equal to the minuend (what gets subtracted from) is inserted at the positive input, and the subtrahend (what is subtracted) is inserted at the negative input. The subtraction operation will take place within the amplifier, and the output will be the result. Fig. 14-3 shows the arrangement.

To multiply a number, the voltage equal to the multiplicand (what gets multiplied) is fed to an amplifier whose gain is equal to the multiplier (what multiplies). The gain is varied by selecting various values of feedback and input resistors. The output will be the input voltage multiplied by the gain. To illustrate, multiply 5 by 10. If 5 V is fed into an amplifier

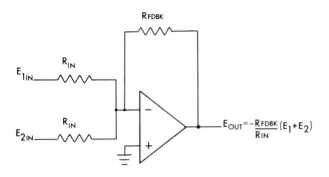

FIG. 14-2.   Operational amplifier as a summer. See text for details.

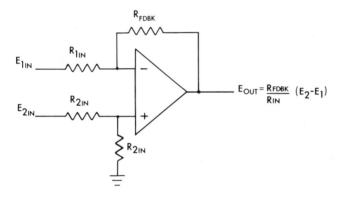

FIG. 14-3.   Operational amplifier as a subtracter. See text for details.

through an input resistor of 10,000 Ω with a feedback resistor of 100,000 Ω, the gain (R_{fdbk}/R_{input}) equals 10; therefore, the output will be 50 V. To divide, the input resistors and feedback resistors are interchanged so that the gain is less than 1. In the example above, the gain of the amplifier would be 1/10, and the output would be equal to 0.5, or 5 divided by 10. This system is useful when the multiplier is a constant, but often the multiplicand and multiplier are variables.

In order to solve problems with multiplicands and multipliers that are variables, logarithms may be used. Recall that to multiply two numbers, their logarithms are added and the antilogarithm of the result will be the product. Some diodes exhibit a logarithmic transfer function, and, if one of these is used in the feedback path of an operational amplifier, the result is a logarithmic gain function for the amplifier. Fig. 14-4 illustrates this. To multiply two variables, they are fed to amplifiers with logarithmic gain functions, summed, and then fed to a final amplifier with an antilogar-

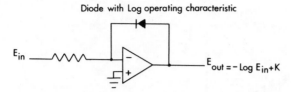

Diode with Log operating characteristic

E_{in}

$E_{out} = - Log\ E_{in} + K$

FIG. 14-4.   Operational amplifier connected in such a way that $E_{out} = \log E_{in}$. See text for details.

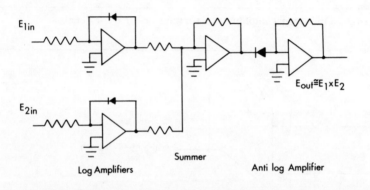

E_{1in}

E_{2in}

$E_{out} \cong E_1 \times E_2$

Log Amplifiers

Summer

Anti log Amplifier

FIG. 14-5.   Instantaneous multiplier operating in real time. See text for details.

ithmic gain function. The output of this final amplifier is the product of the two variables, which continuously changes as the variables change. Fig. 14-5 is an illustration of the system. Notice that in the antilogarithmic amplifier, the diode is at the input and a resistor is in the feedback path, the opposite of the logarithmic amplifier.

The technique described above, using nonlinear elements in the input and feedback circuits, can also result in other gain functions, the square or the cube, for example.

The analog computer is capable of simulating any system for which a mathematical equation can be written. The computer system is relatively easy to arrange, but the mathematical derivation is usually more difficult.

The analog computer consists of 10 to 48 DC amplifiers in a rack or cabinet, with peripheral equipment consisting of the power supplies and controls for setting the initial conditions and for entering the input values. The output can be read from a voltmeter or, in the case of varying signals, from a chart recorder or an oscilloscope. The amplifiers must be stable and low noise. The stability is important for maintaining constant output, and noisy amplifiers would introduce artifacts in the readout.

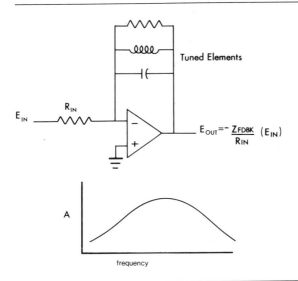

FIG. 14-6.   Operational amplifier connected as tuned amplifier (above). Its transfer function is shown below. See text for details.

As a final illustration of the use of the analog computer, consider the simulation of vowel sounds. Vowels are produced by passing a series of glottal pulses, which resemble a sawtooth wave, through a series of filters formed by the cavities of the vocal tract. To simulate this system, a sawtooth wave is generated by an external signal generator and passed through a series of *tuned amplifiers.* These tuned amplifiers behave like the filter systems set up by the vocal tract cavities. A tuned amplifier and its transfer function are shown in Fig. 14-6. The feedback elements in the amplifier are reactive so that the feedback will vary with frequency. There will be more feedback at some frequencies than at others.

Digital Computers

The modern digital computer is a wondrous device that is already revolutionizing our lives. Conceptually, a digital computer is radically different from an analog computer. The analog computer manipulates voltages whose amplitudes are proportional to some real quantities that the voltages represent or of which they are analogs. The digital computer does not deal with such quantities or qualities. What the digital computer accomplishes is the extremely rapid manipulation of a code, with the code representing anything a programmer chooses it to represent.

Each digital computer incorporates a set or sets of rules for how things are to be coded and for how manipulations on the coded material are to be performed. These sets of rules, which reside in the central processing unit (CPU), relate to a machine language, which is the final set of operating tactics by which the computer carries out the simple switching operations by which it does what it does. The rules in the CPU ensure that the code the programmer desires gets translated properly to the operating level of the machine. The machine language is typically composed and entered into the machine by the manufacturer, and the user is not usually able to manipulate or change it.

The user readies the computer to perform whatever tasks are desired by entering a *program*. A program is a set of instructions to the computer, written in a programming language. The general programming language is also supplied by the manufacturer, but a particular computer task can usually be written in a number of different ways, just as a particular thought can typically be expressed in many different ways. The user constructs a program to carry out some desired task. The program in turn is translated by the machine into a set of steps that the machine can actually carry out. Frequently a small computer's limitations arise from the fact that most of its storage capacity is used in holding the machine language because, in general, the easier a machine is to program, the larger the machine language will be. This limitation may restrict the types of tasks that a small machine can accomplish, although a clever programmer can often work around such limitations. Size limitations are also likely to increase the time taken by the machine to accomplish more complex tasks. The digital computer itself can perform an enormous variety of tasks as long as someone will take the time to encode (program) the task.

As a practical matter, computer technology develops so rapidly that material concerning specific equipment, the control of a computer, and the computer's operation is often out of date before it is even in print. At the same time, much of this background material may be unnecessary in order for the speech therapist to make the best use of computers. Computer programming can be learned by anyone in a relatively short time. This allows the interested person to make use of a computer without knowing anything about the controls on the computer or the electronic operation of the machine. In addition, very little of computer operation is concerned with controls because the majority of the operation takes place in the programming. The goal of this discussion is that the reader obtain some overview of digital computers.

The digital computer can perform all of the operations and simulations of the analog computer, with one exception: it cannot operate in real time. That is, data cannot be processed and printed out as they are received if the data flow is continuous. To circumvent this constraint, data are often recorded, processed at the computer's speed, and then printed out. This constraint prevents complete interaction; that is, it precludes the tabulation of data and the modification of conditions on the basis of changes in the data as they occur. Generally, however, computer speeds are sufficiently high so that the slight delay between input and output while the computer processes the data does not hinder operation in the speech laboratory.

As with the analog computer, if the mathematical statement can be written, the computer can perform the operation. The digital computer can change operating parameters (i.e., the numbers of conditions being manipulated) much faster than the analog because these changes may be written in as part of a program. To change parameters in the analog computer, electronic components must be changed or readjusted. The digital computer can also change parameters in a fixed sequence and graph the output as the parameters change. As an example, Bell Laboratories has programmed a large digital computer to display a cross-section of the vocal tract on an oscilloscope and generate the sound associated with the cross-sectional area that acts as a filter. The computer then changes the sizes of the cavities in an orderly fashion, showing the changes on the oscilloscope and presenting the resultant acoustic signal. In this way, it is possible to observe how a vowel changes character as the lips are gradually parted or the tongue is raised and/or protruded.

The digital computer generates waveforms by constructing the desired shape from a series of discrete values. This allows any of the variables in a wave to be changed in a random or a uniform manner. Much electronic music is generated this way.

In its simplest form, the digital computer consists of a series of on/off switches. All operations and numbers are based on a binary system: either 0 or 1 can exist; the switch is either open or closed. Any external signals fed into the computer must be changed to binary numbers and then, after processing, changed back into decimal numbers for display. The extra steps take time, so the digital computer cannot operate on data instantaneously. (It is interesting to note that computer operation is reaching such high speeds that the length of time it takes for the electrons to travel in the wire is becoming a limiting parameter.)

Early digital computers consisted of a series of toggle switches that could be positioned so that various computations could be performed. Later models used vacuum tubes that operated as switches, and this improved the speed of the computer. Most modern computers operate with solid-state switches. (Experimental models use light or fluid switches.)

Because the information in a computer consists of the presence of a voltage when a switch is closed or the absence of a voltage when a switch is open, these "bits" of information can be stored in several different ways. It is this storage ability that makes the computer so useful.

DIGITAL COMPUTER COMPONENTS

There are many considerations involved in computer selection, but they are best left to a more comprehensive source of information about computers. Let it suffice to say that the computer consists of a *processor,* a *storage device,* and some sort of *terminal* to which information is entered and from which results are read. The output device can be either a television screen or a typewriter. The latter is desirable in that it provides a permanent record, while the former has the advantages of being much faster and conserving paper.

There are two major types of storage devices on all digital computers: *memory* and *mass storage.* The memory is a "black box" that allows immediate access and is used for storing bits while an operation is being performed.

Just a few years ago the device in a digital computer in which information that needed to be retrieved immediately (allowing for the speed of electron flow) was stored was called the *core.* The core was constructed of a series of wires forming a grid. A tiny ring of ferrite was placed at the junction of each vertical wire with each horizontal wire in the grid. If current flowed in both of the wires associated with any given ring of ferrite, that ring would become magnetized. If, at a later time, an instrument that registered the magnetization were connected to the same two wires, the instrument would note that the ring was polarized. By this means, one bit (one small portion of magnetization) could be stored. Imagine thousands of wires forming the grid, resulting in tens of thousands of locations for a ferrite ring, and it is easy to see that quite a large number of bits could be stored in this device. It is also easy to imagine the difficulty of constructing such a device and the expense.

Later developments in computer technology have resulted in semiconductor devices that can perform the same storage operation as the core in much smaller spaces. In addition, the semiconductor devices, unlike the core, can be constructed almost entirely by machine, which results in more precision and less cost. The semiconductor memory devices are generally called just that: *memory.* When we speak of the memory of a computer we are speaking of the core in an older machine and the semiconductor storage device in a newer one, but both the new and old storage devices have almost instant access time. *Almost* instant access time, however, is becoming inadequate for the latest computers, which are called on to perform millions of repetitions of a mathematical operation. Even an access time of a few millionths of a second slows down the process.

The site of the memory often limits the amount of work a computer can perform. Much of the memory will be taken up by the instructions to the computer so that a language may be used, and there may be little room left for data to be entered. The minimal memory size for a smaller computer is 8,000 bits. That means the computer can store the results of the operation of 8,000 separate switches. Computers generally have 16,000- to 64,000-bit memories. Large data processing computers have memories of 1,000,000 bits, or 1 megabit. Experimental models are approaching memory sizes of 1 billion bits, which is still far short of the storage capability of the human cortex, which is estimated to be 4 billion bits.

There are several types of mass storage devices available, and each has its advantages. Magnetic tape is still used on many machines, and its operation is similar to that of the audio machines discussed in Chapter 9, except that only pulses are being recorded. Magnetic tape machines for computer use are expensive and seldom found on laboratory computers. Hard disks, which cost approximately $100 each, are probably the best compromise for a mass storage system. Usually the storage device consists of a disk that is much like a phonograph record but that is housed in a case so that it is not exposed to the air. When the disk is plugged into a machine, a jet of air is continually passed across the record. This keeps the disk clean and also provides a cushion on which the magnetic head rides so that it does not actually touch the disk. The head rides about 50 μ from the surface. The main drawback to disks is the difficulty with keeping them scrupulously clean. Smoke particles, for example, are about 80 μ thick. If one particle comes to rest on the disk and the head attempts to pass over it, there will be a collision, since the head is only 50 μ above the disk. The smoke particle will be ground into the disk and the disk's coating destroyed.

To eliminate this problem, devices called *Winchester disks* have been devised. These contain a disk as before, but in a sealed cabinet. There is no way dirt can enter because the air in the cabinet passes through a filter that eliminates all particles larger than 1 μ. Winchester disk storage devices cost about $500 to $5,000. Some microcomputers use an inexpensive cassette tape player. If the operator already has access to a player, the only additional expense is tape.

The latest storage medium, and one found on most home computers, is the floppy disk. In this system the disk is on flexible plastic and is commonly 5¼ inches in diameter, although other sizes are used. The recording density is not as great as on the hard disk and there is some wear of the head and disk. Both the floppy disk drive and the disk are inexpensive, with the floppy disk costing $1 to $5 each.

The *central processing unit* is the part of the computer in which the operations take place. It is designed so that the operator can issue commands to procure information from storage devices, can accept inputs from various input ports, and can perform mathematical operations on these data. The results are then fed to output ports, from which they are either placed in storage or sent to various display devices. Fig. 14-7 shows a small modern laboratory computer.

The third part of the computer consists of peripheral devices that al-

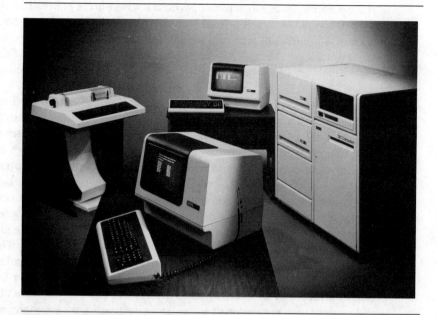

FIG. 14-7.   A laboratory minicomputer adequate for analyzing and synthesizing speech and electrophysiologic signals.

low the computer to interface with other devices. The most common peripheral device is the *keyboard* through which commands can be given to the computer and which eliminates the need to set toggle switches individually. The command functions will be clearer after languages are discussed later in this chapter.

Analog-to-digital (A/D) *converters* are peripheral devices that change analog data, such as a waveform, into digital values that the computer can process. The computer does this conversion to a quality criterion determined by its own complexity. For example, let us consider digitizing a sinusoid. This is done by examining the sinusoid once each time interval, (i.e., quantizing it) and designating its amplitude for that interval. The string of amplitudes is stored as a digital number in the computer, and, when it is desired that the sinusoid be reconstructed, a voltage is generated at each of a string of time intervals, with the voltage being proportional to the stored amplitude. How well a sinusoid is reproduced is determined by the precision of the initial quantizing. For example, if each time interval were infinitely short and each amplitude representation could be any one of an infinite set of values, then the reproduced sinusoid would be an exact replica of the original. The grosser the sampling time and the grosser the amplitude quantization, however, the poorer the stored and reproduced signal. (On the average, the more expensive the computer, the shorter the time sampling and the greater the storage capacity; the larger the number of amplitude steps that can be stored, the better the stored and reproduced sinusoid.) If a sine wave is fed into the computer, the value of the amplitude at each increment of time must be changed into a binary number. The A/D converter does this by measuring the amplitude, converting it into a binary number, and then on command by a timer, repeating the operation. This *sampling* is the factor that slows the computer and prevents real-time operation.

Two kinds of output devices require mention. The first device is the ubiquitous *cathode-ray screen,* which has become familiar through its use in television sets as well as in oscilloscopes. The cathode-ray tube (CRT) displays the instructions, the data, or whatever else has been fed into (inputted) the computer and will also display the results of the operations performed.

Should one desire a more permanent record of the output, then some sort of *printer* is required. Most often the computer will have a printer that provides a permanent output and can print at rapid rates so that the computer's operations are not completely bogged down by the time necessary to print the output. (A large computer facility will often make use of a smaller computer interfaced with the CPU, which serves the function of taking output material from the CPU and feeding it to a printer. In this way, the CPU can dump its output into a smaller computer and go on to process the next batch without having to store the currently unprinted output or to delay its next stages while it awaits the printing operation.) Modern printers print on continuous sheets of paper, but the type is not typically of high quality. The paper is perforated so that it can be separated into single sheets. Most often, even with a minicomputer, one can purchase a high-quality electric typewriter to obtain letter-quality printing under computer control. Often, typewriters with letter-quality printing also allow the use of various sizes of stationery (postcard, standard letter, and so forth).

COMPUTER LANGUAGES

Although the preceding discussion has answered only a few questions concerning the hardware of the digital computer, it must suffice for our purposes. There are many sources of further information listed in the section Suggested Reading.

The secret that allows the non-engineer to use the computer lies with the "high-level" languages, or *software,* that have been devised in the past few years. As we have alluded to previously, the computer performs its operations by having a series of switches open or closed. A specific series of switches is associated with each operation to be performed by the computer. Early computers required the operator to set switches manually, and even today some people prefer to operate computers in this fashion. However, in order to set the proper switches, the operator must understand the logic on which the computer operates and be able to trace its path. This requires a great deal of training and familiarity with computers. Most people using computers today have neither the training nor the time to obtain it; they are usually experts in a discipline other than computers and simply want answers from the computer. Because of this, engineers developed a procedure in which a certain specific pattern of signals could be supplied by a keyboard, with each signal pattern being associated with a specific task for the computer. The keyboard is the standard teletypewriter keyboard.

The next step is the important one for the unsophisticated user to understand: the pattern emanating from the keyboard to the CPU, when the proper word is typed, is the proper signal to make the computer perform an addition. The operator need only learn a language, the words of which are already in the operator's vocabulary. This is a high-level language. FORTRAN, BASIC (one of the easiest), and COBOL are common high-level languages. Each language is designed for specific applications. For example, COBOL is a business-oriented language for keeping records. BASIC is a simple language for performing most mathematical operations.

The simplicity of a language is inversely related to the time and effort taken to develop it. In order to make the language simple for the operator, the engineer must make the operation of the computer very complex. The computer must have stored in its memory the associations between the words typed on the keyboard and the operation to be performed. All this information must be stored so that the computer can quickly decode the word entered and perform the operation. The easier the language is for the user, the more memory space the language will require.

An example of a computer program to add two numbers (A and B), subtract a third number (C), and multiply the result by a fourth number (Z) is illustrated below. The program is written in BASIC. Notice that the language is sufficiently simple that the program can be understood without prior training. More involved operations require a great deal more sophistication, but even these can be learned in a few hours. (Note: The numbers in the left column [10, 20, . . .] are statement numbers and have no function other than keeping the programmer organized. Q, R, and M are arbitrary symbols for values.)

```
10    Enter A
20    Enter B
30    Q = A + B
40    Enter C
50    R = Q - C
60    Enter Z
```

```
70     M = Z × R
80     Print M
90     End
```

The computer used in the speech science laboratory is usually one with one input port, a small memory, and bulk storage capability. This type of computer is called an *interactive computer* because, as the computer processes data, the operator can watch the results and change the parameters. As an example, consider a signal detection task. In this task, the subject will receive a signal via headphones and press a button if the tone is audible. The experimenter can control the intensity, the duration, and the probability of a signal's occurrence by means of typed commands on the teletypewriter. If the subject always responds correctly when the tone is present, the intensity is decreased. When the tone is at an intensity very close to threshold, the subject may be uncertain as to whether or not the tone is present. The subject is told that a correct response results in a monetary reward and an incorrect response results in a penalty. Thus, the probability of the signal influences the decision of the subject to press the button or not because of the value of a correct response and the cost of an incorrect one. For this reason, the experimenter might want to change the probability and is able to do so by changing the program with a typed command. The parameters of the experiment are changed between experimental runs as a function of the responses of the subject who, in turn, is influenced by the costs and values of various responses.

Optional packages of prewritten programs (software packages) are available for laboratory computers. These include programs to operate peripheral equipment, to time the occurrence of internal and external signals, to signal average, to plot the correlation between signals, and to analyze frequency and temporal characteristics of signals. Each of these programs has specific commands that are first fed into the memory. Then commands are typed on the teletypewriter, resulting in various computations and computer functions. These programs are supplied on paper tape or magnetic tape. To use them, the operator loads the program into the memory through the paper tape reader or the magnetic tape reader. The programs have provisions for inserting specific parameters through the keyboard so that the operator can tailor the program to a specific experiment. This software is available at the time the computer is purchased or later.

The *clock function* is one of the most useful peripheral components available for the laboratory computer. It consists of a very accurate timer (accurate to approximately $\pm$ 1 μsec) that generates pulses that can be delivered at rates from about one pulse every 10 seconds to 1,000,000 pulses every second, depending on what rate is selected. The pulses control functions within the computer or within peripheral apparatus connected by cable.

Relays, either electromechanical or solid-state, can be connected to the laboratory computer to control external apparatus. For example, lights can be programmed to switch on and off at rates determined by typed commands. This function is also useful for operating electronic switches to control audio signals in which precise time intervals are necessary.

The flexibility of computer programs is perhaps their greatest advantage. Since experimenters are not always certain of the precise parameters of each experiment, they can write or use flexible programs in which the parameters are varied by typed commands. Otherwise, a specific piece of equipment would have to be used for each task. The program for mathematical computation illustrated earlier is an example. So that any numbers could be used, the commands "Enter A," "Enter B," and so on were used. In this way, the program is changed for each set of numbers. In a program to time a signal, the command "Enter T" could be used. The experimenter would then type in a value for T. To change the timing parameter, only a new value of T need be typed.

Magnetic tape and paper tape devices can also be used to store programs for later use and to store data to be fed in for analysis (paper tape is less often used than magnetic). Most software supplied by computer manufacturers is available on magnetic and paper tape. To program the computer the tape is played and data are taken from the tape and entered into the memory. Direct audio and FM tape machines can also be used for entering data into the computer through the A/D converter. Programs cannot be stored on these machines without modification of the machine and the program.

Currently there is a great deal of talk about microprocessors and devices that are controlled by them. A *microprocessor* is a device that contains some of the same elements as the central processor unit of a digital computer, but the program has been wired into the machine. Consider an audiometer that is "microprocessor-controlled." The microprocessor will determine whether the subject has responded or not, determine whether the attenuation should be increased or decreased, keep track of the threshold, and even select the order of frequency presentation. The microprocessor is a "dedicated" computer. (When a computer or any other device is used exclusively for a single purpose, even though it could be used for a broad variety of applications, it is called *dedicated.*) Some of the advantages of the microprocessor are its freedom from human error, speed and efficiency, and the fact that it can be operated by untrained people. Like all dedicated equipment, the microprocessor has the disadvantages of lacking versatility both within tasks as well as across tasks, becoming dated, and requiring accommodation of people to it rather than of it to people.

Suggested Reading

No references concerning digital computers have been included because they would be superseded by more up-to-date sources many times over by the time this book is published. Your neighborhood librarian or computer center will be happy to recommend the latest guide.

Gilliland, M. C. *Handbook of Analog Computation.* Concord, Calif.: Systron-Donner Corp., 1967.

Johnson, C. *Analog Computer Techniques.* New York: McGraw Hill, 1956.

Malmstadt, H. V., and Enke, C. G. *Digital Electronics for Scientists.* New York: Benjamin, 1969.

Nakatani, L. H. Computer aided signal handling for speech research. *J. Acoust. Soc. Am.* 61:1056–1062, 1977.

VI. Connection

15. Connectors and Connecting

General Considerations

There are one or two important considerations in choosing *plugs,* which are "male" connectors having one or more protruding terminals, as in a standard power cord plug, and *jacks,* which are "female" connectors, such as a standard wall socket, that accept the plug. Very often, however, the designer of a piece of equipment has already made the selection for the user. In general, though, low-level signals such as those obtained in electroencephalographic (EEG) procedures should be connected using plugs that provide the maximum amount of shielding. That is, the braided covering of the cable should be continuous with the outer shell of the plug. For high-frequency signals it is desirable to make certain that the coaxial arrangement of the cable is maintained; that is, the shielding surrounding the signal-conducting cables should retain continuity from plug-end to plug-end for high-frequency signals, and the cables inside the shielding should remain centered so that inappropriate capacitance is not introduced between a conductor and an immediately adjacent shield. Low-impedance circuits with signals at high levels are not prone to picking up interfering levels of induced noise, so the unshielded double banana plug is often used for output to loudspeakers and similar equipment.

MAKING CONTACT

The elements inside the plug slide into receptacles, which means that the connection between plug and receptacle is made by metal sliding on metal. For this reason, the metals used in some receptacles are chosen for their very low electrical resistance. Thus, especially sensitive equipment may have silver contacts since this metal has one of the lowest resistances available. Also, the outer covering of the plug or shield usually provides the ground connection and is often spring-loaded so that when it is attached a spring forces the outer part of the plug against the outer part of the jack. This is one of the principal disadvantages to the RCA pin jack (see Fig. 15-2), as there is no spring loading. Another disadvantage of the RCA pin jack is that it is difficult to remove because of its small size. In laboratory equipment it is desirable to have plugs that can be held firmly while being attached or removed.

MACHINE SCREW CONNECTIONS

Finally, many types of connectors have provisions for connecting the conductors to the terminals by means of machine screws. This means that the wire is held in place by the pressure of the screw against the wire. In a laboratory in which cables are constantly being moved about, it is preferable to solder these terminals in addition to using the screws. In addition, any terminal using screws should have a lock washer under the screw head. The lock washer is simply a circle of metal with sharp points inside or outside the circle. These points have a slight twist to them so that when the screw is tightened the points are bent somewhat. Thus they are constantly pushing out against the screw. This keeps the connections from coming loose because of vibration.

SOLDERING

A word of warning about soldering terminals: soldering consists of heating two pieces of metal so that when a metallic alloy is applied to the two pieces, it melts and coats them. The alloy then plates the two pieces and, since the plating is continuous between both pieces, they are held together. If for any reason there is any corrosion or dirt on either or both of the two pieces of metal, the plating may not take place. The alloy will flow over the surface but will not really fuse with the underlying metal. This is called *cold soldering* and results in a less than adequate junction of the two metals so that there can be a high impedance existing between the elements being joined. For this reason it is extremely important to make certain that both pieces of metal are heated and that the alloy (solder) is melted by the metals being joined and not by the iron doing the heating.

INSULATION

It is also excellent practice to make certain that the insulation on any wire is intact and as close as possible to any connections. The operator will be amazed at how readily conductors throughout a circuit can come into inappropriate contact and short-circuit the signal path.

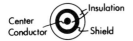

FIG. 15-1.   Cross-section of coaxial cable.

Specifics of Connection

With these general considerations to guide us, let us now consider connectors and connecting in a systematic way.

COAXIAL CABLE

Equipment is connected together by means of *cables.* Plugs on the ends of the cables are inserted into jacks, or sockets, on the various pieces of equipment. *Coaxial cable* is the most common type of cable and is designed to prevent electromagnetic radiation from interfering with the signal. Fig. 15-1 is a cross-section of a coaxial cable. The outer conductor consists of either a braided copper wire or aluminum foil wrapped around the insulation covering the inner conductor. This outer conductor is called the *shield.* It is connected to the equipment "ground" so that if any current is induced in the shield by electromagnetic radiation, it is carried directly to ground and cannot enter the inner conductor, which is the *hot* wire, or that which is carrying the signal from one point to another at a point in the circuit above ground. The inner conductor is either a solid wire or a bunch of fine strands encased in plastic or rubber insulation. Depending on the units being interconnected, there may be more than one conductor inside the shield. For example, if a balanced microphone is being used, there are two wires, one for each side of the microphone. These are insulated from one another, and the shield is the ground. Cables associated with input transducers are small, 20- or 22-gauge wires. For very small devices such as strain gauges, however, the wire may be 24-gauge. In order to make cable flexible, as in microphone cables, the inner cable is made up of many fine wires interspersed with threads called *Litz wire.* The result is a flexible cable, but one which is difficult to solder. If it is necessary to connect these wires, the best practice is to wrap a fine copper wire around the conductor and cover it with solder. Then the conductor can be soldered to plugs or other devices. Ground wires should be heavy, 16- to 18-gauge wire, and connections to earth should be heavy braided cable of 0 or 00 gauge.

A much preferred way of interconnecting equipment with two terminals is to use three-conductor cable consisting of two internal wires and a braided shield. In this case one internal wire connects the two hot terminals; another wire is the common or ground wire; and the shield is connected to ground, *but only at one end.* The shield then isolates the conductors from electromagnetic fields, but does not carry the signal return. The shield should not be connected at both ends because this would result in *two* ground wires, which could result in current flowing between the two ground wires. This undesirable condition, which results in a spurious 60-Hz signal, is called a *ground loop* and should be avoided.

OUTPUT CABLE

Output transducers need heavier wire than input transducers because they carry more current. Coaxial cable is not usually used, because the low impedance of output circuits precludes induced current from stray radiation. Coaxial cable may not be desirable because it can introduce capacitance into the circuit. The capacitance is due to the fact that there are two conductors separated by an insulator throughout the length of the cable. However, at high signal levels this is not usually a problem.

Loudspeakers are best connected with lamp cord of 16- or 18-gauge. This cable will handle several amperes of current without danger of heating or melting.

PLUGS

There is a variety of plugs available for interconnecting electronic equipment, and each type has specific advantages. The scientist is urged to settle on one type of input plug and one type of output plug. This will simplify repair and allow cables to be used for many purposes. Otherwise, it is very difficult to keep track of what goes where. The following paragraphs offer some suggestions to aid in choosing connectors.

Input Plugs

Plugs used with input transducers are constructed so that the inner conductor is enclosed by the ground connection. The shield connects to an outer metal sleeve so that the shielding is continued over the hot lead. This arrangement is apparent from examining the plugs shown in Fig. 15-2. Note also that if there are several inner conductors the plug will have several inner pins. The RCA pin plug is almost universal for interconnection of music systems in ths country. This type of plug is not easy to remove and is difficult to connect, so other types of plugs might be better suited to the laboratory. Other types of plugs shown in Fig. 15-2 can be plugged and unplugged more readily. In addition, they have locking devices so that they cannot become disconnected. The other types also have provisions for clamping the shield to the outer jacket of the cable. This helps to remove much of the strain on the inner connectors should the cable be inadvertently pulled. (Remember to pull on the plug, not the cable, when disconnecting equipment.)

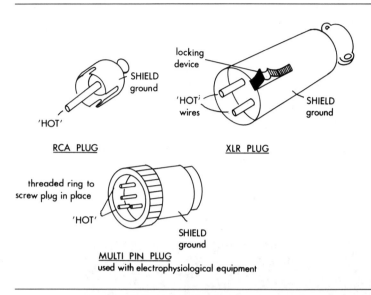

SHIELD ground

'HOT'

RCA PLUG

locking device

'HOT' wires

SHIELD ground

XLR PLUG

threaded ring to screw plug in place

'HOT'

SHIELD ground

MULTI PIN PLUG
used with electrophysiological equipment

FIG. 15-2.   Examples of types of audio plugs.

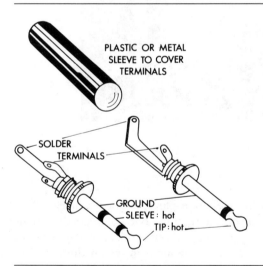

PLASTIC OR METAL SLEEVE TO COVER TERMINALS

SOLDER TERMINALS

GROUND
SLEEVE : hot
TIP : hot

FIG. 15-3.   Three-conductor (left) and two-conductor (right) telephone plugs.

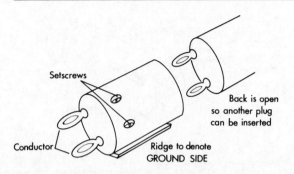

Setscrews

Back is open
so another plug
can be inserted

Conductor

Ridge to denote
GROUND SIDE

FIG. 15-4.   Double-banana output plug.

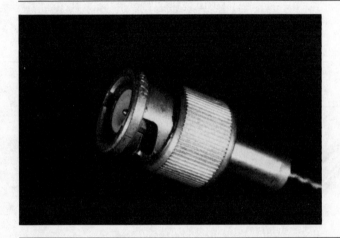

FIG. 15-5.   A BNC plug often used in connected audio apparatus.

Output Plugs

Output plugs are usually telephone plugs, as shown in Fig. 15-3. Two types are shown. The one on the right has two connections, one hot and one ground. The one on the left is a three-conductor plug, which allows connection to a balanced output or input in which there are two hot wires and a ground. Phone plugs can be found with either a plastic cover or a metal cover. The latter provides some shielding and is used with input devices, but it is not necessary with output devices. Besides the phone plug, the other type of output plug commonly found is the *double-banana* (Fig. 15-4). This type of plug allows stacking; that is, several devices may be connected to the same point. An example is the connection of a voltmeter across a loudspeaker, both of which are connected to the output of a power amplifier. The wires are not soldered, but held in place by setscrews. This is handy when interchanging wires, but the set-screws often loosen. Note that the double-banana is polarized so that the ground wire is always connected to the side with the ridge. Caution must be used so that this side is always connected to the ground side of the circuit. If it is connected backward, it is possible to short circuit the output device, which can result in burnt transistors and worse. Other types of output plugs are manufactured by various companies, but these are the most common. The BNC plug shown in Fig. 15-5 is common in broadcast work and audio.

VII. Application of
Basic Principles

16. Analysis of Instrumental Needs

This chapter examines clinical problems and the equipment needed to address them in situations that involve the application of what has been learned. As the reader will see, the approach to solving these problems consists of (1) a statement of what is clinically desired, (2) consideration of the desired output from the equipment as a means of identifying the specific instrumentation need, (3) one or more systems for accomplishing the desired instrumental task, and (4) comments on particulars that the clinician needs to consider. We expect that you will have the satisfaction of following the examples with some ease and will develop some skill in understanding the preliminary analyses that lead to determining what equipment you require for a clinical or research task. We begin by returning to the examples that began the book.

Assessment of Hypernasality

The first example concerns the client who has undergone surgical repair of a palatal cleft. The speech and language pathologist is asked to make some judgment concerning hypernasality. The first method of assessment would require the client to speak a passage repeatedly while the clinician listens carefully. As Fig. 16-1 shows, the ear listening to the talker must have sufficient fidelity (and training) to hear nasal emission. There are obvious shortcomings to this technique: client fatigue, variation in speech repetitions, limited speech sample. The second choice would be to use a tape recorder as shown in Fig. 16-2. Here the same constraints apply to the microphone as to the ear in the first example.

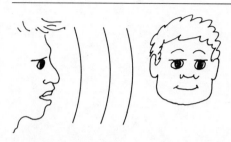

FIG. 16-1.   The simplest method of analysis of nasal emission.

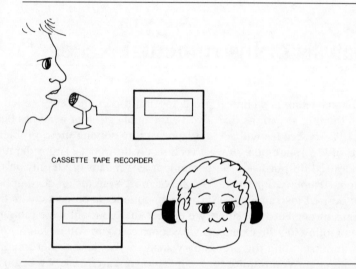

CASSETTE TAPE RECORDER

FIG. 16-2.   A method of speech analysis that permits repeated assessment.

The third choice is shown in Fig. 16-3 where the sound spectrograph allows the clinician to visualize the intensity of the various frequencies present during an utterance. Again, the quality of the microphone is important. Also, it may be necessary to adjust the compression circuit within the spectrograph so that the weak, high frequencies receive additional amplification.

Notice that all the techniques described thus far relate to the acoustic signal, which is directly influenced by the presence or absence of nasality. Because it would appear more efficient to look at nasality directly, the pneumotachograph is the fourth instrumental choice. The pneumotachograph is shown in use in Fig. 16-4 (see also Chap. 12). It is a closed system for capturing the air emitted from the nose or mouth or both and measuring its volume velocity (the analog in the acoustic domain of electrical current). The important characteristics of the system are that its

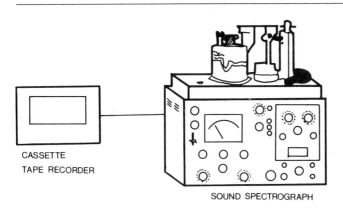

FIG. 16-3.   A relatively precise method of acoustic speech signal analysis.

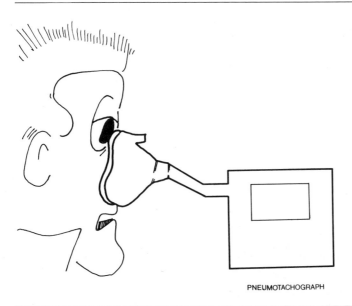

PNEUMOTACHOGRAPH

FIG. 16-4.   The pneumotachograph, which provides a quantified assessment of nasal emission.

input matches the impedance of open space so that the vocal system does not alter its characteristics because a measuring system is coupled to it, and the instrument must be capable of an accurate measure of either the relative oral-to-nasal emission or the absolute emission, depending on the question. In our present example, only a relative measure is needed.

Assessment of Vocal Strain

The second example involves the man experiencing vocal strain that, in the clinician's preliminary impression, is caused by too low a habitual pitch. The clinician's approach to the problem is to prescribe a weekend of vocal rest and then to record the man's lowest and highest sustainable pitches and a sample of his habitual speaking voice. She requires first a tape recorder/reproducer with a microphone and reel of tape.

Her diagnostic tactic derives from her knowledge from voice science about the expected level of optimal pitch within one's own vocal range. She will use this knowledge to help locate the desired pitch level to which therapy will be directed, provided she proves correct that his habitual pitch is too low and therefore the likely cause of the vocal strain.

Four alternatives exist for the pitch analysis: an oscilloscope, a digital computer, a sound spectrograph, or a direct pitch-reading device. We will consider the use of each piece of equipment in turn.

The oscilloscope is used by taking a sample of the lowest sustained pitch, making a continuous tape loop from a portion of the sample and reproducing the portion continuously as input to the vertical amplifier. The horizontal amplifier is used to display time, and, as has been discussed, the horizontal amplifier is calibrated in time. The fundamental frequency repetition rate of the low-pitched sample can be read from the oscilloscope, and this "pitch period" can be converted to frequency (frequency [f] in cycles per second equals 1 second divided by the time per cycle; $f = 1/\text{period}$). The fundamental frequency of the highest sustainable tone can likewise be obtained from a tape-recorder loop, as can the frequency of a sample of recorded speech. In the case of the recorded speech, because the vocal pitch will vary during the sample, obtaining a reasonable pitch estimate becomes a statistical, or sampling, problem. The sampling problem is outside our discussion because it has to do only with how many samples are evaluated and not with how the evaluation is done.

The second scheme uses a digital computer to accomplish the same analytic tasks. The particular scheme used in programming the computer may vary with the size and capacity of the machine and the skill and sophistication of the programmer. The most common technique, called *Fourier analysis,* is based on a mathematical theorem that states that any wave can be analyzed into some fundamental frequency plus overtones. The machine simply executes these mathematical steps on each waveform in turn, in each case deriving some fundamental voice pitch. One alternative procedure is for the computer program to match the waveform to successively earlier portions of itself, that is, to do an autocorrelation so as to find its own fundamental repetition rate and to calculate fundamental frequency from this periodicity.

The third scheme requires making a sound spectrograph and reading the fundamental pitch directly off the graph by using a calibrated scale; the fourth method uses one of the commercially available devices designed and dedicated to direct derivation of vocal pitch (e.g., the Visipitch). The Visipitch is an instrument manufactured by Kay Elemetrics Corporation (Pine Brook, N. J.) that consists of a microphone connected to a processor built into an oscilloscope. When a trigger on the side of the microphone is depressed, a beam begins to travel across the face of the oscilloscope. The vertical position of the beam is determined by either the pitch or the intensity of the voice, or both, selected by a switch on the face of the instrument. Because the oscilloscope is a storage machine, the trace is displayed on the face of the oscilloscope until an erase button is depressed, which clears the screen.

Whichever analytic scheme is used, the analysis is accomplished and the man's habitual vocal pitch determined. If the clinical hypothesis of too low a habitual pitch is validated, therapy would be initiated and progress could be charted by measuring the client's ability to achieve and maintain use of a higher vocal pitch and the reduction and cessation of his vocal strain.

Assessment of Muscular Tension

Our third example is more closely allied to a laboratory study than the previous two. A student suggests that, when subjected to delayed auditory feedback (DAF), she experiences a tightening of her facial muscles, which, she believes, results in some change in vocal quality. She desires to test the first half of her hypothesis by using electromyographic (EMG) recordings of her facial muscles under normal reading and DAF reading.

EXPERIMENTAL DESIGN CONSIDERATIONS

As is true with any experiment, a variety of decisions are required. We will concern ourselves only with those directly related to the instrumentation issues. They are:

1. The environment within which the EMGs will be taken
2. The muscles from which potentials will be taken
3. The choice and placement of electrodes and the instrument to record the EMG signals
4. The choice of microphone, tape deck (with DAF capability), tape, and headphones
5. The amount of DAF and the signal level of the fedback speech

Some of the research considerations we are ignoring are:

1. The sample size (single or multiple subjects)
2. The selection of material to be read

3. The determination of the criterion level for the EMG: What magnitude of change is necessary to validate the hypothesis (e.g., average EMG, peak value during an utterance, total integrated EMG during a reading, peak value on key words)?

The first consideration is the EMG environment. Electromyographic signals, picked up by surface electrodes, are of levels no higher than many stray electrical fields. Ideally, therefore, the subject and the electrode pick-up should be shielded from stray fields. Frequently, EMG recording is done in copper-shielded sound suites (audiometric suites), where the copper shield around the room is connected to an earth ground so as to protect the internal environment from stray electromagnetic fields.

If such a space is not available, one can try placing the equipment and subject in a variety of locations, seeking ones that appear not to be subjected to large amounts of radiation. One way to do this is to hook up all equipment, including the EMG electrodes, and measure the magnitude of signal in the electrode pick-ups with and without a human subject present. The location giving the largest difference in signal level for the presence of the subject is the location of choice.

There are several obvious considerations in making the choice of muscles to be monitored. In order of importance, they are: the muscles must be representative of the desired behavior, easily accessible, and smooth and flat enough to be able to accept electrodes. In the present case, let us assume that we have decided to place disk electrodes on the buccal (cheek) surface, 1 inch posterior and 1 inch superior to the corner of the mouth in repose. The instrument we will use is a multiple-channel EEG machine typically used in the hearing and speech center for doing brainstem evoked audiometry.

The tape deck of choice may be a machine with record and playback heads especially designed for DAF; that is, the spacing between these heads (the delay) can be continuously varied. If such a machine is not available, the minimum requirement is a tape deck allowing the listener to monitor under earphones either the signal to the recording head or the signal from the playback head; in addition, the signal must be controlled by a switch so that the subject can switch from the one signal to the other rapidly and easily. The microphone characteristics are relatively unimportant since the fidelity of the recording is not at issue. The same is true of the choice of tape and of headphones. Obviously, the microphone and headphones must be properly matched to the tape deck in impedance, so that a reasonable signal level can be attained. The feedback level to the listener should be set to the most comfortable loudness in the undelayed condition. If the amount of delay is variable, the examiner may choose to experiment with a few settings to find one that seems to interfere with normal speech rhythm maximally.

The study is then conducted using the magnitude of the EMG in the normal feedback and the delayed feedback conditions to test the student's hypothesis about facial muscle tightening under delay.

Assessment of Airflow

The next example concerns an effort to answer a question about the pressure and amount of air flowing during speech and so involves assessing two phenomena. The first phenomenon is the total airflow during an utterance, and the other is the changes in intraoral pressure during the utterance. The latter is obtained by examining the moment-to-moment changes in intraoral pressure, and the former is the integrated total of these instantaneous values through the time of the utterance.

It will be necessay to capture all the air expired during the speech, so the subject(s) will wear a mask, similar to those used for respirators, to which a pneumotachograph will be attached. The pneumotachograph, as discussed earlier (see also Chap. 12), is a closed system containing an acoustic resistance and a pressure transducer sensitive to the pressure changes across the resistance. The pressure change across the resistance is equivalent to the volume velocity of air through the resistance, so the instantaneous pressure change plus the integrated or total value are the two measures required.

OPERATION OF THE EQUIPMENT

There are some practical considerations in using this equipment. The acoustic resistance is typically a tapered tube of many inches. This tube requires support, usually a microphone boom, to prevent its weight from pulling the mask loose. The mask itself must be tight enough to capture all the expired air but not so tight as to restrict articulatory movement. The differential pressure transducer requires a polarizing voltage, so adjustments are necessary in order to center the indicator on the recording device. Most often the pressure transducer is connected to a multichannel electrophysiologic recorder.

The transducer is connected to its preamplifier, and the appropriate switch is set to provide the necessary polarizing voltage. The recording unit will have a switch labeled *voltage/pressure* or something similar. In the voltage position, the input is connected differentially to the input amplifier. In the pressure position, the input connections are the same, but a polarizing voltage is supplied through two additional wires in the cable to the transducer.

We first set the switch to the pressure position. The preamplifier gain is set low and the control on the amplifier labeled *zero adjust* is moved to position the pen in the middle of the recording chart. The preamplifier gain is then increased, and the zero adjust on the preamplifier is adjusted to return the pen to the middle of the chart. This latter adjustment varies the polarizing voltage across the transducer so that the output voltage is zero when the diaphragm is at rest. During data collection this adjustment is frequently necessary because differential transducers drift. Check it often.

The intraoral pressure is measured using a pressure transducer connected to a piece of vinyl tubing that is then placed in the mouth at the back of the oral cavity. The tubing is made of small-diameter, thin-walled plastic, similar to the kind used with aquarium aerators. It is placed between the cheek and lower teeth and hooks around the last molar as shown in Fig. 16-5. The electrical adjustment with this transducer is the same as the differential.

When the subject now speaks with the transducers in place and adjusted, the result is similar to Fig. 16-6. The upper trace is the instantaneous volume velocity, and the lower is the intraoral air pressure.

A measure of the total airflow is required, so the output of the pneumotachograph amplifier is fed to an integrator. An integrator consists of a high-gain amplifier with a capacitor as the feedback element. The capacitor accumulates and stores the voltage appearing at the input. The integrator is an optional component with most electrophysiologic recorders. After passing through the integrator, the recording appears as in Fig. 16-7. The lower trace is the integrated voltage, which represents the total air expired. After recording each utterance, the capacitor must be discharged by short circuiting it with a switch or a relay. The integrator reset button performs this operation.

Troubleshooting

If one of the traces is missing and the others are correct, interchange the preamplifiers. If the missing trace moves, the trouble is a defective preamplifier. If the trace does not move, interchange transducers. If the trace now moves, the associated cable could also be defective. The cables connecting pressure transducers are small and fragile and most likely to break at the end where they are inserted into the plug or the transducer. A technician should repair this problem. If the trace does not move, the trouble is localized to the power amplifier or the galvanometer. If the power amplifiers can be interchanged, try that. If the trace moves, the trouble is a defective power amplifier. If the trace does not move, it is the galvanometer or the cable connecting it to the power amplifier. Note that in all the foregoing discussion it is assumed that if the problem seems to be associated with the interoral pressure transducer, the operator first has made certain that the tubing is not collapsed or blocked with saliva.

The output of the integrator can appear to be quite erratic if the preamplifier and amplifier are not zeroed very carefully. If there is a slight DC voltage present at the output of the preamplifier because of a zero

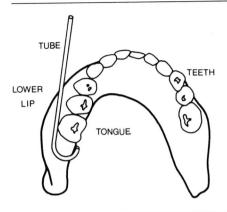

FIG. 16-5. Tube for measuring intraoral air pressure.

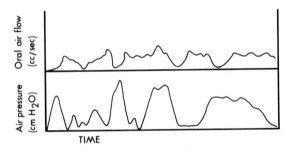

FIG. 16-6. Oral airflow (above) and intraoral air pressure (below) during an utterance.

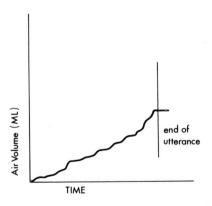

FIG. 16-7. Total airflow recording (from integrator).

imbalance, this DC voltage will be integrated and cause the integrator pen to move even in the absence of a transducer signal.

Assessment of Cortical Potential

Students taking a course in stuttering phenomena hear a report concerning the *contingent negative variation* (CNV) *phenomenon* and decide to observe it while it is occurring. The CNV phenomenon is a slow negative DC shift of the electroencephalographic (EEG) signal that is considered to be anticipatory activity prior to some motoric activity. It appears to maximize after approximately 3 seconds and to continue for some few seconds beyond its peak. The students hypothesize that CNV is more likely to occur in moments of dysfluency than during fluent speech, so they opt to obtain measures on some speech considered dysfluent and some considered fluent.

The phenomenon is measured using a surface electrode placed on the vertex (the vertex is the junction of the coronal and temporal sutures), with a negative lead clipped onto one earlobe and a ground to the other. The cortical signal is fed to an analog-to-digital (A/D) converter, digitizing it so that it can be fed into a digital computer for storage and analysis. In a typical procedure, the subject hears and immediately repeats recorded passages.

EXPERIMENTAL DESIGN CONSIDERATIONS

The experimental and equipment setup is somewhat more complicated than that encountered previously, so let us consider the conceptual needs of the study.

1. The data must be in a form that a digital computer can accept and analyze.
2. The subject must hear a recorded passage and then repeat it. No data can be gathered during playback, but data collection must begin immediately following the playback.
3. Data collection must occur only during the several seconds following passage playback.
4. Analysis must differentiate data into the two classes: fluent response and dysfluent response.
5. Data in each class must be averaged so that the result tests differences in amount of CNV occurrence in the two classes.

Let us deal with each of the conceptual needs in turn to arrive at an appropriate laboratory setup. The signal arriving at the digital computer that must be stored and evaluated is in the form of a continuous voltage waveform (an EEG). A digital computer requires a signal of some one of a number of specified magnitudes, and it can accept only one signal in a given (but very short) time period. Therefore, the incoming signal must be digitized, which is accomplished by the A/D converter. The A/D converter accepts a voltage input for some sampling period and, at the end of the period, delivers a single-valued voltage to the computer while accumulating the input voltage from the next sampling period. The digital computer's storage capacity and program allow, for example, any of 64 amplitude values or any of 512 amplitude values. The single-valued voltage delivered to the computer can be only one of these acceptable values, so the stored value may be some small distortion of the actual input value. Obviously, the fewer amplitude values the computer can accept and the longer the storage period, the poorer will be the stored representation of the original voltage wave impinging on the A/D converter. The data arising from the EEG electrodes on the subject and digitized by the A/D converter can enter a storage bank in the computer for further processing, but there are only certain time periods during which data gathering is appropriate. The CNV phenomenon occurs in the moments following a signal that causes the subject to anticipate motor activity, in this case the beginning of his repetition of the recorded passage. The EEG data germane to the occurrence, if at all, of the CNV are gathered in the time immediately following delivery of the prerecorded passage to the subject. Therefore, what is desired is some process that will suppress data generation during the delivery of the recorded passage and initiate data collection immediately as the passage ends. Further, because the CNV is a short-term phenomenon, economy of data collection is advanced if the prerecording is "chunked" into separate short segments, such as 10 seconds each, with each segment separated by some additional 10 seconds to allow CNV data acquisition.

Our proposal for a data suppression/data release circuit uses a computer program that behaves like a Schmitt trigger. A Schmitt trigger is an electrical circuit that supplies a pulse when triggered. In this instance the circuit is triggered by the output of the tape-reproducing system that stores the recorded passages, and the computer is programmed so that no EEG information is accepted while the trigger pulse is present. The effect is that, while the subject is hooked up to electrodes and the signals are transmitted to the A/D converter and thence to the computer, EEG data are gathered only during the period following presentation of the recorded passages. That is, data are gathered only during and immediately following the expected occurrence of the CNV.

The next instrumental issue is classification of EEG information into two groups of signals, those associated with fluent speech and those associated with dysfluent speech. This decision to differentiate fluent from dysfluent speech might be argued in some cases, but the laboratory implementation is independent of the criteria used, and a suggested procedure is as follows: let us feed the EEG data into a temporary storage bank and program the computer to move the data into the pool labeled *dysfluent speech* if a Schmitt trigger pulse is delivered within 3 seconds or to move the data into the pool of *fluent speech* if no pulse is delivered. We then give a push button to the experimenter with the instruction that the button is to be pressed if the speech is dysfluent. The push button supplies an input to a Schmitt trigger program within the computer.

The EEG analysis process, for both of the classes, makes use of the unpredictability of moment-to-moment EEG variation and the predictability of the slow negative DC shift that is the CNV. Because the EEG signal is seemingly random in its voltage polarity and magnitude, and if an average is taken over an appreciable time, the average output tends toward zero since the positive and the negative values tend to cancel one another out.

Except for the CNV, the averaged EEG data pool for either the fluent or dysfluent speech should approach zero output. The CNV will influence this output by superimposing a negative DC, hypothesized by the students to be greater during dysfluent than fluent speech.

OPERATION OF THE EQUIPMENT

The subject has the electrodes applied as discussed earlier and is seated in a comfortable chair in front of a loudspeaker. The electrodes are connected to the physiologic amplifier, and the output of the amplifier is connected to the A/D converter of the computer. The tape-recorder output is connected both to the power amplifier supplying the loudspeaker and to a Schmitt trigger on the computer. A recorded passage is played and the subject immediately responds. The recorded passage triggered the signal-averaging program in the computer, and the EEG data are stored in the core. When the subject completes a response, the experimenter decides whether the subject is fluent or dysfluent. If the latter, the button is pushed and the computer program causes the averaged data to be stored in the dysfluent memory. If the button is not pressed, the data are stored in the fluent memory. After 20 or 30 passages, the computer program causes the data to be printed out on the teletype or, better yet, graphed on the oscilloscope. The oscilloscope record is stored by taking a photograph of the screen. A camera is an optional accessory that fits over the face of the oscilloscope screen. If a storage oscilloscope is available, it is possible to trace the image on the screen on onionskin paper.

TROUBLESHOOTING

No EEG Signal

If the output of the amplifier shows no activity, check for power to the unit. The electrode leads may be short circuiting against one another. The cable to the computer from the amplifier may be defective. If an oscilloscope is available, connect the amplifier output directly to the oscilloscope. If all the amplifier switches are set correctly and there is still no signal, the amplifier is probably defective. In assessing the CNV, the highpass filter should not be in the circuit because the signal of interest is a DC and any filtering will prevent its observation. The lowpass filter is set at 5 Hz to eliminate other EEG signals.

Erratic EEG Signal

The presence of spurious signals is most often caused by poor contact of one or more electrodes. The resistance between electrodes should be less than 10,000 Ω. Movement of the electrode leads can cause erratic signals, so the leads should be taped to the subject's head or neck so they cannot flex. The amplifier balance should be checked frequently. The amplifier drift often appears similar to the CNV.

No Averaged Signal

Incorrect temporal parameters can cause the CNV to be obscured. If the averaging begins too early, the CNV is never seen. If the averaging begins too late, only the recovery phase may be seen. These are not equipment problems and are beyond the scope of the book, but the experimenter is urged to make use of the literature to define the temporal parameters of any EEG experiment before attempting to examine the data. Incorrect averaging times often appear to be equipment problems.

Suggested Reading

Note: Books dealing with specific pathologies will also refer to instrumental techniques.

Borden, G. J., and Harris, K. S. *Speech Science Primer.* Baltimore: Williams & Wilkins, 1984.

Geddes, L. A., and Baker, L. E. *Bio-medical Instrumentation.* New York: Wiley, 1968.

Lass, N. J. (Ed.). *Contemporary Issues in Experimental Phonetics.* New York: Academic, 1976.

Lehiste, I. (Ed.). *Readings in Acoustic Phonetics.* Cambridge, Mass.: MIT Press, 1969.

Lieberman, P. *Speech Physiology and Acoustic Phonetics: An Introduction.* New York: Macmillan, 1977.

Luchsinger, R., and Arnold, G. E. *Voice-Speech-Language.* Belmont, Calif.: Wadsworth, 1965.

Mackay, R. S. *Biomedical Telemetry.* New York: Wiley, 1970.

Minifie, F. D., Hixon, T. J., and Williams, F. *Normal Aspects of Speech, Hearing and Language.* Englewood Cliffs, N. J.: Prentice-Hall, 1978.

Perkell, J. S. *Physiology of Speech Production.* Cambridge, Mass.: MIT Press, 1969.

Peterson, H. A., and Marquardt, T. P. *Appraisal and Diagnosis of Speech and Language Disorders.* Englewood Cliffs, N. J.: Prentice-Hall, 1981.

Venables, P. H., and Martin, I. *Manual of Psychophysiological Methods.* New York: Elsevier, 1967.

Watkins, K. L., and Zagzebski, J. A. On-line ultrasonic technique for monitoring tongue movement. *J. Acoust. Soc. Am.* 54:544–547, 1973.

17. Analysis of Common Equipment

Pure-Tone Audiometer

The construction of a piece of equipment or pieces of complementary equipment to fulfill a particular set of laboratory or clinical conditions can be illustrated in many ways. Perhaps the most commonly found examples are associated with the equipment used in audiologic assessment, so let us use some of this equipment as a basis for a variety of tasks. We will consider what the components of an audiometer should be, how they are sequenced (i.e., the logic of the audiometer's construction), and critical points in determining the audiometer's quality and ease of operation, including its calibration.

An audiometer is a device that delivers any of a variety of signals to the auditory system, allowing the user to specify the level at which the signal is delivered. Its components include signal sources, transducers, amplifiers for increasing signal levels, calibrated variable resistors (attenuators) for increasing or decreasing input or output levels by controlled amounts, and meters or other designators of signal level.

If we take the simple case of a discrete-frequency, pure-tone, air- and bone-conduction audiometer, we can describe the basic necessities of an audiometer and subsequently elaborate on the more complex machines.

THE COMPONENT PARTS

Fig. 17-1 is a block diagram of the elements in a pure-tone audiometer. There are really only a few components necessary for its construction. They are (1) an oscillator, (2) tuning circuits for the oscillator, (3) amplifier, (4) compensation networks for the level to each headphone (and

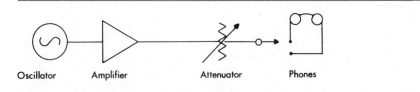

Oscillator   Amplifier   Attenuator   Phones

FIG. 17-1.   Block diagram of a pure-tone audiometer.

to the bone oscillator), and (5) the hearing loss attenuator. The oscillator is at the left-hand side of Fig. 17-1 and is composed of an active element (or two) with tuned networks that control the frequency. To change the frequency, the operator moves a switch that determines the tuned components connected to the oscillator. If a given frequency is not accurate, the tuned components can be replaced on the board inside the audiometer. The output of the oscillator is then passed on to an amplifier that drives the headphones.

The amplifier in the audiometer must be an extremely good one because the dynamic range requirements are so large—120 dB at some frequencies. There must also be a very low noise level, and various types of amplitude distortion must be less than 0.1%. Following the amplifier are several compensation networks that allow the engineer to match the headphones at each of the test frequencies. There are three boards with solder terminals present, one associated with each of the headphone channels and one associated with the bone oscillator channel. The terminals of the boards are specific to the test frequencies, so it is only necessary to measure the sound pressure level (SPL) output and adjust it to the proper value at each frequency and with each output transducer by soldering a resistor of the proper value to the associated terminals. The frequency selection switch also connects the output of the amplifier to various terminals of the calibration boards because different amounts of amplification are necessary at each frequency due to the headphone response. Some more complex audiometers, and especially the large clinical speech audiometers that also have pure-tone capability, replace the terminal boards with variable resistors so that calibration can be done by adjusting the resistor with a screwdriver.

Finally, the attenuator is connected at the output just prior to the headphones. This connection results in the best signal-to-noise ratio, as discussed in Chapter 3.

The normal ear, like any other physical device, shows a variable response to frequency. As we know, the ear is most sensitive to a band in the middle of its response range (i.e.,1,000–4,000 Hz) and is less sensitive to frequencies above and below this middle band. For convenience, however, we prefer to consider hearing loss as a decrement in sensitivity of some greater or lesser amount (i.e., as a threshold shift of such and such an amount), no matter what frequency. Therefore, we use a scale (hearing threshold level) so conceived that zero is the normal or expected value and any loss is expressed as a deviation from this norm. The need to adjust the output of each frequency generator to the appropriate level to represent normal sensitivity for that frequency is an additional reason for having independent level-setting capability for each frequency. Another switch is required to channel the output to the selected transducer (the earphone plus the cushion coupling the earphone to the ear).

Because the human auditory system comprises two ears, it is possible to deliver a signal to one ear that is of a sufficiently high level that it can be heard by the other. If the ears are closely matched in sensitivity, then the significantly greater loudness in the tested ear will mask the sound's presence in the opposite ear. However, if the tested ear has a significant decrement in sensitivity, then the sound may be heard in the opposite (better) ear before the level of the sound reaches the zero in the ear under test. The subject will respond, and the examiner will mistakenly conclude that the tested ear has better hearing than it really does. This problem is avoided by providing a masking noise, of some known level, to the better ear. A discussion of the characteristics of the masking noise and of the designation of appropriate level(s) is not germane here, but note that an audiometer requires a masking noise that can be specified by level and frequency characteristics and that is automatically channelled to the non-test ear when needed.

While Fig. 17-1 schematizes a pure-tone audiometer, the device shown is not operational because it lacks an interruptor switch. The *interruptor switch* in most audiometers performs a more complex function than simply turning the signal on and off. First, it is often desirable for the clinician to choose whether the signal should be normally off and turned on by the switch, or normally on and turned off by the switch. In many audiometers, the clinician has the option of choosing either, which results in yet another switch to reverse the action of the interruptor switch. Second, since the ear is particularly sensitive to signal changes, the turning on and turning off of a pure tone must be done with some care or the listener may become aware of the clicks generated by the switching even though he or she is not able to hear the tone itself at the level at which it is delivered.

In addition, there are some design and construction particulars about an audiometer that relate to the interface of technical and human factors. For example, do the electrical construction and circuit layout facilitate maintenance and repair (e.g., are plug-in circuits used)? Are calibration potentiometers and variable reactors labeled? Does the user's manual or technical manual facilitate local repair or must the unit be returned to the factory? Are components reasonably available or must they be specially fabricated and available only on special order?

Obviously, the individual who is relatively unsophisticated in electronics and laboratory instrumentation will be less confident about making construction and design decisions. It is helpful to make a side-by-side comparison of several audiometers, if possible, when attempting to evaluate their quality and ease of use. At that same time, examination of the interiors of each machine will likely show up differences in the care taken in circuit layout and construction.

CALIBRATION PROCEDURES

The American National Standards Institute (ANSI) has developed a standardized system for calibrating audiometers, giving the standards to be met and allowable variances. Let us now consider the rationale underlying calibration without a concern for the specific levels required by the appropriate standard.

The calibration of an audiometer ensures adequate performance of the equipment for the tasks we have built it to perform: (1) to deliver any of a series of tones, (2) at any of a wide range of output levels, (3) to either of the subject's ears. The tester must be able (4) to turn the tone on and off without the subject being aware of the change, other than by hearing the tone. The problem here is that when a switch is activated an instantaneous surge of energy, called a *transient,* may occur. A transient is perceived as a click and contains a broad band of frequencies much like a white noise. For this reason an audiometer interruptor turns a tone on gradually over a 5-10-millisecond time to prevent transients, (5) to alter the level of tonal output by known amounts, and (6) to mask out the non-test ear so that the test is not invalidated by cross-hearing.

The calibration procedures must include measures of (1) the frequency and purity of frequency content of the tone, (2) the fidelity of the output attenuator, (3) the independence (isolation of the two channels or the lack of cross-talk) of the two earphone circuits, (4) the envelope-shaping introduced by the tone interruptor switch, (5) the overall level at some specified output, and (6) the quality (frequency content) of the masker, its overall level at some specified output, and the linearity of the masker attenuator.

Calibration requires a device that couples a headphone to the calibration instrumentation so that a measurement is made from the actual acoustic output, which, in normal testing, is the stimulus to the subject. That device in turn must connect to a frequency analyzer for measures 1 and 6 above, to a time control and display system (such as an oscilloscope) for measure 4, and to a voltmeter for measures 2, 3, and 5. The standards to be met in a calibration of a pure-tone audiometer are detailed in an ANSI publication, numbered ANSI S3.6-1969 (R1973).

Speech Audiometer

The same principles and system involved in the calibration of a pure-tone audiometer apply to the calibration of a speech audiometer. A speech audiometer is a device for delivering any of a variety of signals (live voice, recorded speech, noise, or any of an assorted variety of complex sounds) to either ear under earphones at a known presentation level or to either or both of a pair of loudspeakers such that the signal level at the listener's ear is known and specifiable. Its components include (1) a microphone, (2) a noise generator, (3) a tape deck and phonograph table, (4) an arm and cartridge for reproducing recorded signals, (5) a meter (or meters) to establish the signal level for material varying in level, (6) variable-level input resistors to adjust signal input level, (7) an amplifier for each channel, (8) variable-level output resistors to adjust the output level to be delivered to the final transducers, (9) switching systems for signal selection and for output transducer selection, and (10) transducers.

The audiometer should also have a feedback channel from patient to clinician, which consists of a microphone, amplifier, and transducer with a variable resistance for setting listening level. While the feedback system requires good fidelity and a reasonable dynamic range, it need not be calibrated for sound pressure level.

The set of specifications for calibrating the audiometer must include criteria for frequency response range, dynamic amplitude range and allowable distortion by the microphone, any other input signal transducer, the earphones and the loudspeakers, the amplifiers in the system, and the characteristics of the noise generator. Short-term variability in spectrum and long-term frequency stability must be specified. The tolerance of the volume controls (potentiometers or attenuators) must be specified for each setting.

The Tape Recorder/Reproducer

As yet another illustration of how our needs translate to equipment specifications, let us explore a common situation. I find that my daily activities would be facilitated if I carried a small tape cassette machine, so I decide to buy one. My major purpose is to be able to make oral notes for later entry into client records, my daily log, and the like. My criteria, therefore, are that the machine produce intelligible speech, be relatively economical, be battery operated, and be portable.

Then I decide that perhaps I would like to record an occasional meeting. My additional criteria are, then, that the machine have a nondirectional microphone and greater signal sensitivity (to pick up both near and far voices). Then I decide that I may also want to do occasional dictation. My additional criteria are that the machine have a precise start-stop mechanism, editing control, location-finder, and built-in mechanics for remote control (to allow foot-pedal operation during transcription). I next decide that perhaps I would like to record an occasional client. My additional criteria are that the machine have a good frequency response to microphone and loudspeaker (good low-frequency response for voice quality, vocal pitch, and the like, and good high-frequency response for precision of articulation and the like; the microphone must allow recording of both lows and highs, and the loudspeaker must be able to reproduce both).

Finally I decide that I may want to use the machine for recording concerts. My additional criteria are that the machine have a superior tape-drive mechanism to control flutter (moment-to-moment rapid variations in tape speed and, therefore, in pitch, coming about because of mechanical components being slightly out-of-tune) and wow (slower variations than flutter in tape speed causing slowly varying changes in pitch). In addition, the machine must have lower distortion in the electronics and greater dynamic range than a recorder for speech alone, because music will reveal distortion more readily than speech because music may have more than twice the dynamic range.

The example can be further elaborated, but we can sum up here. For the first use, an adequate cassette machine can probably be purchased for less than $50. But the cost of the machine will rapidly increase with each additional set of requirements, and will greatly increase if we shop for a machine for high-quality music recording. The primary lesson to be gleaned from this rather lengthy discussion is that one needs to first specify the uses to which the equipment will be put, then the characteristics of the signals to be processed and the requirements for the ultimate output, and finally the dimensions of the signals being processed. With these specifications in hand, the prospective purchaser need only examine the specifications of possible units and buy the one that meets the requirements at the minimum price. A final caveat: Never accept a machine's published specifications without question. Always measure the performance of the equipment and, if it does not meet the specifications that convinced you to purchase it, return it posthaste.

Edinburgh Masker

The Edinburgh masker has an unusual combination of circuit elements. The device was designed because of the suggestion that presenting a sawtooth masking signal to a speaker's ear might prevent dysfluency while that person is speaking.

An Edinburgh masker thus requires (1) a device to generate a signal

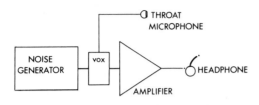

FIG. 17-2.   Block diagram of an Edinburgh masker.

to be fed to an earpiece and (2) a means to switch the generator on only when the user speaks. The masking signal comes from a sawtooth signal generator. The generator is connected to an amplifier that terminates in an earpiece. The amplifier has an added circuit at its input called a voice-operated relay (VOX). The VOX is a device that will not allow a signal to pass through it until a voltage is presented to a "switching input." When a voltage is present at the switching input, the VOX is closed and a signal can pass from the signal input to the signal output.

In the Edinburgh masker, a throat microphone supplies the switching input so that when the speaker begins phonation, the masker is turned on. The masking noise ceases whenever the speaker stops. Fig. 17-2 shows the arrangement.

Instrument Design

There are a great many types of "dedicated" equipment—equipment that is designed to perform one task to the exclusion of all other tasks. Nevertheless, with the background the student has obtained thus far in reading this book, it should be possible to guess how some dedicated equipment is designed. The following examples are our guesses concerning how a few devices might operate, based on our knowledge of instrumentation. In no case have we any more information than the name of the unit, the advertising material, and a quick look at the device at a convention of the American Speech, Language and Hearing Association. Certainly the actual equipment will operate more efficiently than the designs contained herein, if only because the engineers designing the equipment have built prototypes and spent countless hours "debugging" the prototype (*debugging* is removing errors in the operation of a device).

The first example concerns a device that indicates when a talker has uttered an /s/ that is distorted, with its sound approximating the /sh/. This distortion usually indicates that additional high frequency energy is present. The first requirement for our detector is an input transducer to change the spoken acoustical signal into an electrical signal. Then this signal will be amplified. Next, there must be a device to determine if there is high-frequency energy present. This would be a highpass filter tuned to the range in which the distorted /s/ would occur. The output of the filter would then be fed to another amplifier with a lamp at its output. If the filter passes only the unacceptable frequencies, the lamp will light only when unacceptable frequencies are present in the signal. The amplifier output might be fed to a self-latching relay so that if the distorted sound occurs the lamp will be lighted and stay that way until turned off. A self-latching relay circuit might be desirable because the duration of the faulty signal might be so short that the observer would fail to detect it. There are also meters that hold and indicate a peak reading until reset.

Consider a system that shows the presence or absence of various bands of frequencies. That is, particular sounds have certain frequency patterns that allow them to be distinguished from other sounds. If a system is constructed with a series of filters, the outputs of which are connected to various colored lamps, the result is a device that will convert an acoustic spectrum into a visible spectrum. This means that various sounds will have lights associated with them due to the acoustic spectra. Fig. 17-3 shows a block diagram of the device. The possible number of filters is unlimited. The various colored lamps and their associated filters and driven amplifiers can be arranged in a stack from low frequencies to high or in any other arrangement that seems logical. The gain controls are set to such positions that a particular sound will show a logical visible pattern. (One particularly important reason for the gain controls is that there is less energy in the higher frequencies of speech so that additional amplification must be made for the spectra of various speech sounds even before any phoneme differentiation is done.)

Another simple example of a dedicated device is a device that indicates nasal sound emission. The unit uses a contact microphone or an accelerometer. The contact microphone is really just a rather insensitive microphone that is equipped with a diaphragm that is placed on, or interfaces with, a vibrating surface instead of interfacing with the air. If the surface moves, the diaphragm moves and a current is generated. An accelerometer functions in the same way. In any case, the microphone or accelerometer is placed against the side of the nose. If sound passes through the nose, the tissue will vibrate. The resultant movement generates an electrical signal in the transducer that is fed to an amplifier and thence to the indicating device. The gain control is necessary because even non-nasal sounds cause some minimal movement of the tissues of the head. Another more complicated but more useful system would consist of an airflow transducer that is coupled to the nares so that when air passes through the nares, the indicating device is triggered. If another airflow transducer is coupled to the oral cavity and the outputs of the transducers are fed to an analog computer so that the ratio of the two

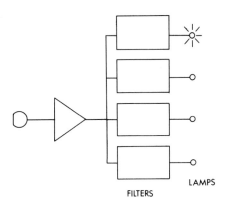

FILTERS   LAMPS

FIG. 17-3.   Schematic of spectrally associated light display.

outputs is computed, the result provides the oral/nasal ratio, which some have found to be important in assessing velar sufficiency.*

As a screening device, a threshold detector might be included so that if the oral/nasal ratio is below a certain value (meaning that there is more than normal nasal flow), an indicating device is triggered. So far as we know the latter device has not been marketed.

In any situation in which a variable signal is to operate a switch, it is necessary to remove most of the variation in the wave. To illustrate this, consider the wave in Fig. 17-4. This could be a speech signal. If one wanted that signal to operate a timer so that vocalization time could be measured, for example, it would be desirable to smooth out the signal so that the timer would not be triggering off and on for each individual wave. The circuit usually used for this is called the Schmitt trigger. A Schmitt trigger is an amplifier that conducts maximally as soon as an input signal exceeds an adjustable threshold (see following examples). The device does not conduct until the threshold is exceeded, and then conducts at its maximum. Thus, if a speech signal were fed into the trigger, the output might appear as in Fig. 17-5. To refine the circuit further, lowpass filtering is added so that the unit does not trigger between peaks. The result is a wave as in Fig. 17-6. The unit will operate when the threshold is exceeded and will continue to stay on as long as the input does not drop below the frequency for which the filter is set. For speech, this could be somewhere in the neighborhood of 75 Hz.

The Schmitt trigger is ubiquitous and is the heart of many common laboratory devices. As can be seen from the figures, it does remove much

*Shelton, R. L., Knox, A. W., Arndt, W. B., and Elbert, M.   The relationship between nasality scale values and oral and nasal sound pressure levels. *J. Speech Hear. Res.* 10:549, 1967.

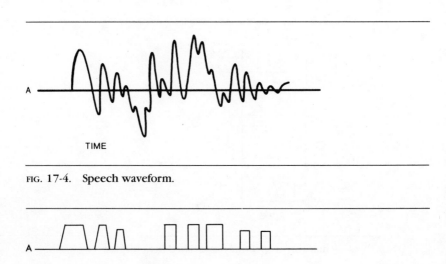

FIG. 17-4. Speech waveform.

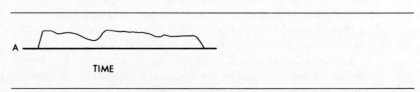

FIG. 17-5. Waveform of Fig. 17-4 after passing through Schmitt trigger.

FIG. 17-6. Waveform of Fig. 17-5 after lowpass filtering.

of the microstructure of the wave, which may not be of any importance in the processing at hand. For example, if one were attempting to measure the fundamental frequency of a speaker, the high-frequency perturbations would only further confound the measurements, so the signal is often fed through a Schmitt trigger. The lowpass filter would be eliminated in this case so that the fundamental would not be filtered out.

Finally, consider a device, one of several types currently on the market, for treatment of vocal intensity disorders. Some devices are constructed to provide a visual or auditory signal when the user's vocal intensity is too loud and others provide a visual or auditory signal when it is too weak. Other units can be set to perform either function. This should be relatively easy to visualize as a device that has a microphone, probably a throat microphone or contact microphone that can be taped to the tissue near the larynx, and an amplifier whose output goes to a switch that turns on a light or sounds a signal. The unit that signals when the intensity is too loud is controlled by a gain control on the amplifier. When the input to the amplifier exceeds a level selected by the microphone wearer, a switch is operated. This switch will probably be a relay, and the

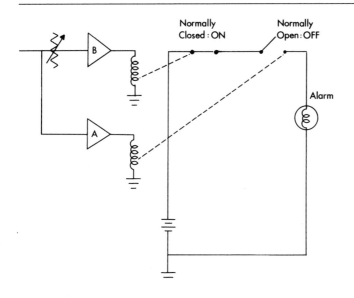

FIG. 17-7.   Electromechanical signal system for voice intensity.

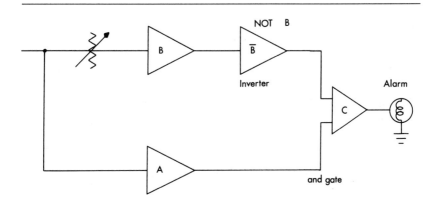

FIG. 17-8.   Digital logic system for voice intensity signal.

relay can be connected to turn on several lights or perform a multitude of other functions.

The circuit that signals when the vocal intensity is too weak would be a little more complex, but might appear as in Fig. 17-7 or Fig. 17-8. These two figures illustrate two different methods of control, one called *electromechanical control* and the other called *digital logic control.* Fig. 17-7 shows the output of two amplifiers connected to relays. The relay to amplifier A is switched on any time there is an input to amplifier A, (i.e., whenever the subject speaks). Amplifier B switches its relay off any time the input exceeds a selected level. This level is chosen and the sensitivity of the amplifier is adjusted with the gain control. Thus, if the level to amplifier B exceeds the threshold, the relay will be switched off and the circuit to the lamp will be broken. If, however, the level is not sufficiently loud to trigger the relay, the circuit through the warning light is completed and it signals that the subject is not speaking louder than the threshold to amplifier B. This is the electromechanical system that can be duplicated by the digital logic of Fig. 17-8. In this case, the output of both amplifiers is fed to Schmitt triggers. Thus, if the level to the amplifier exceeds a specific threshold level, the output of the Schmitt trigger reaches its maximum. The unit at C is called an AND gate, which switches only when both inputs to the unit are at a maximum. If the subject is speaking, the input at A is at the maximum. If the level of speech is above the threshold of trigger B, the output is maximum. Now comes the unusual part of this circuit: the output of B is fed to an inverter that has a maximum output when the input is minimum and vice versa. In this case, the input is maximum so the output is minimum. This is fed to an AND gate, but the AND gate cannot fire because one input is at a maximum and the other is at a minimum. Thus, the warning light stays off because the input level was sufficient. If the level was insufficient to trigger B, the output would be at the minimum, the output of the inverter would be at the maximum, and the two inputs to the AND gate would be equal, so the gate would fire and the warning light would come on.

The foregoing description of a digital logic circuit serves only to introduce the topic and to acquaint the reader with the general subject. Digital logic is being used in many circuits, but it is being rapidly supplanted by microcomputers, which can duplicate all of the digital logic functions and also allow an almost infinite variation of the parameters. This allows the designer to change the circuit without having to obtain other logic elements; the microprocessor duplicates all the circuits needed.

Appendix

Attenuators

The *attenuation* or loss introduced by an attenuator is defined as the ratio in decibels of the power delivered by the source into the attenuator circuit to the power delivered by the attenuator into the load, when the load matches the attenuator output in impedance (i.e., when the attenuator load "sees" or is terminated in its image impedance). Let us, after McElroy,* call this power ratio k^2; thus, k^2 = power into attenuator/power into load, and the attenuator loss = $10 \log k^2 = 20 \log k$.

The following equations provide adequate information for designing attenuators to suit most applications in the speech and hearing science laboratory. These equations are optimized for the minimal loss resulting from slight mismatches of the input and output impedances. Obviously some compromises have been made, and there may still be further slight mismatches due to the tolerance of resistors that are used in the circuits.

Unbalanced Network Attenuators

T-NETWORK ATTENUATOR

Perhaps the simplest attenuator that we will consider is the T-network, or T-pad, which is an example of an unbalanced attenuator (Fig. A-1). The T-pad consists of three resistors, each of which must be variable so that each can be set at precisely the required value to achieve an impedance match for the source, another match for the load, and some desired value of attenuation.

The conditions that we have established for the attenuator are (1)

*Designing resistive attenuating networks. *I. R. E. Proc.:* March 1935.

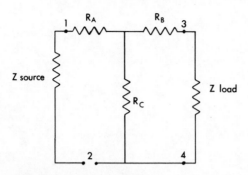

FIG. A-1. T-pad schematic.

some source impedance (R_s) to be matched by the attenuator, (2) some load impedance (R_L) to be matched by the attenuator, and (3) some desired attenuation (k^2). The conditions that we must satisfy are (1) the impedance at terminals 1 and 2 with R_L connected must equal R_s, (2) the impedance at terminals 3 and 4 with R_s connected must equal R_L, and (3) the power delivered into terminals 1 and 2 must be k^2 times the power at R_L.

These conditions give rise to three equations (see McElroy), which factor to:

$$R_A = R_s \left(\frac{k^2 + 1}{k^2 - 1} \right) - 2 \sqrt{R_s R_L} \left(\frac{k}{k^2 - 1} \right)$$

$$R_B = R_L \left(\frac{k^2 + 1}{k^2 - 1} \right) - 2 \sqrt{R_s R_L} \left(\frac{k}{k^2 - 1} \right)$$

$$R_C = 2 \sqrt{R_s R_L} \left(\frac{k}{k^2 - 1} \right)$$

McElroy presented tables of various values of the attenuation factor as it is used in varieties of attenuators. Table A-1 is one such table.

The T-pad formula for a network between equal impedances follows. This pad serves to present a constant impedance to both source and load as well as to introduce some predetermined attenuation. In the equal impedance case, $R_A = R_B$ and $R_s = R_L$. The formulas are:

$$R_A = R_B = R_s \left(\frac{k - 1}{k + 1} \right)$$

$$R_C = 2R_L \left(\frac{k}{k^2 - 1} \right)$$

TABLE A-1. Constants for attenuator equations

n(db)	$r = \dfrac{1}{k}$	k	k^2	$\dfrac{k-1}{k+1}$	$\dfrac{k+1}{k-1}$	$\dfrac{k}{k^2-1}$	$\dfrac{k^2-1}{k} = k - r$	$\dfrac{k^2+1}{k^2-1}$	$\dfrac{k-1}{k} = 1 - r$	$\dfrac{k}{k-1} = \dfrac{1}{1-r}$	$\dfrac{1}{k-1} = \dfrac{1}{rk-1}$	n(db)
0.05	0.994260	1.0057731	1.011579	0.0028783	347.43	86.8618	0.011513	173.73	0.0057395	174.22	173.22	0.05
0.1	0.98855	1.011579	1.023292	0.0057562	173.73	43.4303	0.023029	86.866	0.011448	87.363	86.363	0.1
0.2	0.97724	1.023292	1.047128	0.011512	86.866	21.713	0.046052	43.437	0.022762	43.933	42.933	0.2
0.3	0.96605	1.035143	1.071520	0.017268	57.911	14.473	0.069093	28.965	0.033949	28.455	28.455	0.3
0.4	0.95499	1.047128	1.096477	0.023022	43.437	10.854	0.092138	21.730	0.045007	22.219	21.219	0.4
0.5	0.94406	1.059254	1.12202	0.028774	34.754	8.6810	0.11519	17.391	0.055939	17.877	16.877	0.5
0.6	0.93325	1.071520	1.14815	0.034525	28.965	7.2327	0.13827	14.499	0.066746	14.982	13.982	0.6
0.7	0.92257	1.083928	1.17490	0.040274	24.830	6.1974	0.16136	12.435	0.077428	12.915	11.915	0.7
0.8	0.91201	1.096477	1.20227	0.046019	21.730	5.4209	0.18447	10.888	0.087988	11.365	10.365	0.8
0.9	0.90157	1.10917	1.23027	0.051763	19.319	4.8168	0.20760	9.6853	0.098429	10.160	9.1600	0.9
1.0	0.89125	1.12202	1.25893	0.057502	17.391	4.3335	0.23077	8.7237	0.10875	9.1954	8.1954	1.0
1.1	0.88105	1.13051	1.28825	0.063237	15.814	3.9376	0.25396	7.9384	0.11895	8.4069	7.4069	1.1
1.2	0.87096	1.14815	1.31826	0.068968	14.499	3.6076	0.27719	7.2842	0.12904	7.7499	6.7499	1.2
1.3	0.86099	1.16145	1.34896	0.074695	13.388	3.3283	0.30046	6.7313	0.13901	7.1939	6.1939	1.3
1.4	0.85114	1.17490	1.38038	0.080418	12.435	3.0888	0.32376	6.2579	0.14886	6.6176	5.7176	1.4
1.5	0.84139	1.18850	1.41254	0.086132	11.610	2.8809	0.33711	5.8480	0.15861	6.3050	5.3050	1.5
1.6	0.83176	1.20227	1.44544	0.091846	10.888	2.6991	0.37051	5.4899	0.16824	5.9439	4.9439	1.6
1.7	0.82224	1.21618	1.47911	0.097551	10.251	2.5384	0.39394	5.1744	0.17776	5.6258	4.6258	1.7
1.8	0.81283	1.23027	1.51356	0.103249	9.6853	2.3956	0.41744	4.8944	0.18717	5.3427	4.3427	1.8
1.9	0.80353	1.24452	1.54882	0.108939	9.1794	2.2676	0.44099	4.6442	0.19647	5.0897	4.0897	1.9
2.0	0.79433	1.25893	1.58489	0.11463	8.7241	2.1523	0.46460	4.4195	0.20567	4.8620	3.8620	2.0
2.2	0.77625	1.28825	1.65959	0.12597	7.9384	1.9531	0.51200	4.0322	0.22375	4.4692	3.4692	2.2
2.4	0.75858	1.31826	1.73780	0.13728	7.2842	1.7867	0.55968	3.7108	0.24142	4.1421	3.1421	2.4
2.5	0.74989	1.33352	1.77828	0.14293	6.9966	1.7133	0.58363	3.5698	0.25011	3.9983	2.9983	2.5
2.6	0.74131	1.34896	1.81970	0.14856	6.7313	1.6457	0.60765	3.4399	0.25829	3.8657	2.8657	2.6
2.8	0.72444	1.38038	1.90546	0.15980	6.2579	1.5245	0.65594	3.2088	0.27556	3.6289	2.6289	2.8

TABLE A-1 (continued)

n(db)	$r = \dfrac{1}{k}$	k	k^2	$\dfrac{k-1}{k+1}$	$\dfrac{k+1}{k-1}$	$\dfrac{k}{k^2-1}$	$\dfrac{k^2-1}{k} = k-r$	$\dfrac{k^2+1}{k^2-1}$	$\dfrac{k-1}{k} = 1-r$	$\dfrac{k}{k-1} = \dfrac{1}{1-r}$	$\dfrac{1}{k-1} = \dfrac{1}{r^{-1}-1}$	n(db)
3.0	0.70795	1.41254	1.99526	0.17100	5.8480	1.4192	0.70459	3.0095	0.29205	3.4240	2.4240	3.0
3.2	0.69183	1.44544	2.08930	0.18215	5.4899	1.3269	0.75361	2.8360	0.30817	3.2450	2.2450	3.2
3.4	0.67608	1.47911	2.18776	0.19326	5.1744	1.2453	0.80302	2.6838	0.32392	3.0872	2.0872	3.4
3.5	0.66834	1.49623	2.2387	0.19879	5.0304	1.2079	0.82789	2.6147	0.33166	3.0152	2.0152	3.5
3.6	0.66069	1.51356	2.2909	0.20432	4.8944	1.1725	0.85289	2.5493	0.33931	2.9472	1.9472	3.6
3.8	0.64565	1.54882	2.3988	0.21532	4.6442	1.1072	0.90314	2.4298	0.35435	2.8221	1.8221	3.8
4.0	0.63096	1.58489	2.5519	0.22627	4.4194	1.0483	0.95393	2.3229	0.36904	2.7097	1.7097	4.0
4.5	0.59566	1.67880	2.8184	0.25340	3.9464	0.92323	1.08314	2.0999	0.40434	2.4732	1.4732	4.5
5.0	0.56234	1.77828	3.1623	0.28013	3.5698	0.82241	1.21594	1.9249	0.43766	2.2849	1.2849	5.0
5.5	0.53088	1.88365	3.5481	0.30643	3.2633	0.73922	1.35277	1.7849	0.46912	2.1317	1.1371	5.5
6.0	0.50119	1.99526	3.9811	0.33228	3.0095	0.66932	1.49407	1.6709	0.49881	2.0048	1.0048	6.0
6.5	0.47315	2.1135	4.4668	0.35764	2.7961	0.60964	1.6403	1.5769	0.52685	1.89807	0.89807	6.5
7.0	0.44668	2.2387	5.0119	0.38246	2.6146	0.55801	1.7920	1.4985	0.55332	1.80730	0.80730	7.0
7.5	0.42170	2.3714	5.6234	0.40677	2.4584	0.51291	1.9497	1.4326	0.57830	1.72918	0.72918	7.5
8.0	0.39811	2.5119	6.3096	0.43051	2.3228	0.47309	2.1138	1.3767	0.60189	1.66142	0.66142	8.0
8.5	0.37584	2.6607	7.0795	0.45366	2.2043	0.43765	2.2849	1.3290	0.62416	1.60216	0.60216	8.5
9.0	0.35481	2.8184	7.9433	0.47622	2.0999	0.40592	2.4636	1.2880	0.64519	1.54993	0.54993	9.0
9.5	0.33497	2.9854	8.9125	0.49817	2.0074	0.37730	2.6504	1.2528	0.66503	1.50368	0.50368	9.5
10.0	0.31623	3.1623	10.000	0.51950	1.9249	0.35137	2.8561	1.2222	0.68377	1.46247	0.46247	10.0
10.5	0.29854	3.3497	11.220	0.54026	1.8512	0.32775	3.0512	1.1957	0.70146	1.42559	0.42559	10.5
11.0	0.28184	3.5481	12.589	0.56026	1.7849	0.30616	3.2663	1.1726	0.71816	1.39245	0.39245	11.0
11.5	0.26607	3.7584	14.125	0.57969	1.7251	0.28635	3.4923	1.1524	0.73393	1.36253	0.36253	11.5
12.0	0.25119	3.9811	15.849	0.59848	1.6709	0.26811	3.7299	1.1347	0.74881	1.33545	0.33545	12.0
12.5	0.23714	4.2170	17.783	0.61664	1.6217	0.25127	3.9799	1.1192	0.76286	1.31085	0.31085	12.5
13.0	0.22387	4.4668	19.953	0.63416	1.5769	0.23568	4.2429	1.1055	0.77613	1.28845	0.28845	13.0
13.5	0.21135	4.7315	22.387	0.65105	1.5360	0.22123	4.5202	1.0935	0.78865	1.26799	0.26799	13.5

14.0	0.24926	1.24926	0.80047	1.0829	4.8124	0.20780	1.4985	0.66733	25.119	5.0119	0.19953
14.5	0.23208	1.23208	0.81164	1.0736	5.1204	0.19529	1.4642	0.68298	28.184	5.3088	0.18836
15.0	0.21629	1.21629	0.82217	1.0653	5.4456	0.18363	1.4326	0.69804	31.623	5.6234	0.17783
15.5	0.20175	1.20175	0.83212	1.0580	5.7887	0.17275	1.4035	0.71250	35.481	5.9566	0.16788
16.0	0.18834	1.18834	0.84151	1.0515	6.1511	0.16257	1.3767	0.72639	39.811	6.3096	0.15849
16.5	0.17595	1.17595	0.85038	1.0458	6.5338	0.15305	1.3519	0.73970	44.668	6.6834	0.14962
17.0	0.16449	1.16449	0.85875	1.04071	6.9382	0.14413	1.3290	0.75246	50.119	7.0795	0.14125
17.5	0.15387	1.15387	0.86665	1.03621	7.3655	0.13577	1.3077	0.76468	56.234	7.4989	0.13335
18.0	1.14402	1.14402	0.87411	1.03220	7.8174	0.12792	1.2880	0.77637	63.096	7.9433	0.12589
18.5	1.13488	1.13488	0.88115	1.02866	8.2950	0.12055	1.2698	0.78755	70.795	8.4139	0.118850
19.0	1.12638	1.12638	0.88780	1.02550	8.8003	0.11363	1.2528	0.79823	79.433	8.9125	0.112202
19.5	1.11847	1.11847	0.89407	1.02269	9.3347	0.10713	1.2369	0.80844	89.125	9.4406	0.105925
20.0	1.11111	1.11111	0.90000	1.02020	9.9000	0.10101	1.2222	0.81818	100.000	10.0000	0.100000
20.5	0.10425	1.10425	0.90559	1.01799	10.498	0.095255	1.2085	0.82747	112.202	10.5925	0.094406
21.0	0.097845	1.09875	0.91087	1.01601	11.131	0.089841	1.1957	0.83634	125.893	11.2202	0.089125
21.5	0.091870	1.09187	0.91586	1.01426	11.801	0.084739	1.1837	0.84478	141.254	11.8850	0.084139
22.0	0.086291	1.08629	0.92057	1.01270	12.510	0.079935	1.1726	0.85282	158.49	12.589	0.079433
22.5	0.081070	1.08107	0.92501	1.01126	13.260	0.075411	1.1621	0.86048	177.83	13.335	0.074989
23.0	0.076190	1.07619	0.92921	1.01007	14.054	0.071148	1.1524	0.86777	199.53	14.125	0.070795
23.5	0.071623	1.07162	0.93317	1.00897	14.895	0.067133	1.1432	0.87470	223.77	14.962	0.066834
24.0	0.067345	1.06734	0.93690	1.00799	15.786	0.063348	1.1347	0.88130	251.19	15.849	0.063096
24.5	0.063339	1.06334	0.94043	1.00712	16.728	0.059778	1.1267	0.88756	281.84	16.788	0.059566
25.0	0.059584	1.05958	0.94377	1.00634	17.727	0.056413	1.1192	0.89352	316.23	17.783	0.056234
25.5	0.056066	1.05607	0.94691	1.00565	18.783	0.053238	1.1121	0.89917	354.81	18.836	0.053088
26.0	0.052762	1.05276	0.94988	1.00504	19.903	0.050246	1.1055	0.90455	398.11	19.953	0.050119
26.5	0.049665	1.04966	0.95268	1.00449	21.088	0.047422	1.0993	0.90965	446.68	21.135	0.047315
27.0	0.046757	1.04676	0.95533	1.00400	22.342	0.044757	1.0935	0.91448	501.19	22.387	0.044668
27.5	0.044026	1.04403	0.95783	1.00356	23.672	0.042245	1.0881	0.91907	562.34	23.714	0.042170
28.0	0.041461	1.04146	0.96019	1.00317	25.079	0.039874	1.0829	0.92343	630.96	25.119	0.039811
28.5	0.039052	1.03905	0.96242	1.00283	26.569	0.037636	1.0781	0.92755	707.95	26.607	0.037584
29.0	0.036786	1.03679	0.96452	1.00252	28.149	0.035526	1.0736	0.93147	794.33	28.184	0.035481

TABLE A-1 (continued)

n(db)	$r = \frac{1}{k}$	k	k^2	$\frac{k-1}{k+1}$	$\frac{k+1}{k-1}$	$\frac{k}{k^2-1}$	$\frac{k^2-1}{k} = k - r$	$\frac{k^2+1}{k^2-1}$	$\frac{k-1}{k} = 1-r$	$\frac{k}{k-1} = \frac{1}{1-r}$	$\frac{1}{k-1} = \frac{r}{1-r}$	n(db)
29.5	0.033497	29.854	891.25	0.93518	1.0693	0.033534	29.821	1.00225	0.96650	1.03466	0.034657	29.5
30.0	0.031623	31.623	1,000.0	0.93869	1.0653	0.031655	31.591	1.00200	0.96836	1.03266	0.032655	30.0
31.0	0.028184	35.481	1,258.9	0.94518	1.0580	0.028207	35.453	1.00159	0.97182	1.02900	0.029001	31.0
31.5	0.026607	37.584	1,412.5	0.94817	1.0547	0.026627	37.558	1.00142	0.97339	1.02733	0.027334	31.5
32.0	0.025119	39.811	1,584.9	0.95099	1.0515	0.025135	39.786	1.00126	0.97488	1.02577	0.025766	32.0
33.0	0.022387	44.668	1,995.3	0.95621	1.0458	0.022398	44.646	1.00100	0.97761	1.02290	0.022900	33.0
34.0	0.019953	50.119	2,511.9	0.96088	1.04072	0.019961	50.099	1.00080	0.98005	1.02036	0.020359	34.0
34.5	0.018836	53.088	2,818.4	0.96302	1.03840	0.018843	53.069	1.00071	0.98116	1.01920	0.019198	34.5
35.0	0.017783	56.234	3,162.3	0.96506	1.03621	0.017788	56.216	1.00063	0.98222	1.01810	0.018105	35.0
36.0	0.015849	63.096	3,981.1	0.96880	1.03221	0.015853	63.080	1.00050	0.98415	1.01610	0.016104	36.0
37.0	0.014125	70.795	5,011.9	0.97214	1.02866	0.014128	70.781	1.00040	0.98588	1.01433	0.014328	37.0
37.5	0.013335	74.989	5,623.4	0.97368	1.02703	0.013338	74.976	1.00036	0.98666	1.01352	0.013516	37.5
38.0	0.012589	79.433	6,309.6	0.97513	1.02550	0.012591	79.420	1.00032	0.98741	1.01275	0.012750	38.0
39.0	0.0112202	89.125	7,943.3	0.97781	1.02270	0.0112216	89.114	1.00025	0.98878	1.01135	0.011348	39.0
40.0	0.0100000	100.00	10,000.	0.98020	1.02020	0.0100010	99.990	1.00020	0.99000	1.01010	0.010101	40.0
40.5	0.0094406	105.925	11,220.	0.98130	1.01906	0.0094414	105.916	1.00018	0.99056	1.00953	0.0095306	40.5
41.0	0.0089125	112.202	12,589.	0.98233	1.01799	0.0089134	112.193	1.00016	0.99109	1.00899	0.0089926	41.0
42.0	0.0079433	125.89	15,849.	0.98424	1.01601	0.0079436	125.88	1.00013	0.99206	1.00801	0.0080070	42.0
43.0	0.0070795	141.25	19,953.	0.98594	1.01426	0.0070795	141.24	1.00010	0.99292	1.00713	0.0071301	43.0
43.5	0.0066834	149.62	22,387.	0.98672	1.01346	0.0066834	149.61	1.00009	0.99332	1.00673	0.0067286	43.5
44.0	0.0063096	158.49	25,119.	0.98746	1.01270	0.0063096	158.49	1.00008	0.99369	1.00635	0.0063496	44.0
45.0	0.0056234	177.83	31,623.	0.98887	1.01131	0.0056234	177.83	1.00006	0.99438	1.00566	0.0056551	45.0
46.0	0.0050119	199.53	39,811.	0.99003	1.01007	0.0050119	199.53	1.00005	0.99499	1.00504	0.0050370	46.0
46.5	0.0047315	211.35	44,668.	0.99058	1.00951	0.0047315	211.35	1.000045	0.99527	1.00475	0.0047540	46.5
47.0	0.0044668	223.87	50,119.	0.99111	1.00897	0.0044668	223.87	1.000040	0.99553	1.00449	0.0044869	47.0
48.0	0.0039811	251.19	63,096.	0.99207	1.00799	0.0039811	251.19	1.000032	0.99602	1.00400	0.0039970	48.0

49.0	0.0035607	1.00356	1.000025	0.99645	281.84	0.0035481	1.00712	0.99293	79,433.	281.84	0.0035481	49.0
50.0	0.0031723	1.00317	1.000020	0.99684	316.23	0.0031623	1.00634	0.99370	100,000.	316.23	0.0031623	50.0
51.0	0.0028264	1.00283	1.000016	0.99718	354.81	0.0028184	1.00565	0.99438	125,890.	354.81	0.0028184	51.0
52.0	0.0025182	1.00252	1.000013	0.99749	398.11	0.0025119	1.00504	0.99499	158,490.	398.11	0.0025119	52.0
54.0	0.0019992	1.00200	1.000008	0.99801	501.19	0.0019953	1.00400	0.99602	251,190.	501.19	0.0019953	54.0
55.0	0.0017815	1.00178	1.000006	0.99822	562.34	0.0017783	1.00356	0.99645	316,230.	562.34	0.0017783	55.0
56.0	0.0015874	1.00159	1.000005	0.99842	630.96	0.0015849	1.00317	0.99684	398,110.	630.96	0.0015849	56.0
57.0	0.0014145	1.00141	1.000004	0.99859	707.95	0.0014125	1.00283	0.99718	501,190.	707.95	0.0014125	57.0
58.0	0.0012605	1.00126	1.000003	0.99874	794.33	0.0012589	1.00252	0.99749	630,960.	794.33	0.0012589	58.0
60.0	0.0010010	1.00100	1.000002	0.99900	1,000.0	0.0010000	1.00200	0.99800	10^6	1,000.0	0.0010000	60.0
65.0	0.00056265	1.00056	1.000001	0.99944	1,778.3	0.00056234	1.00112	0.99888	3.1623×10^6	1,778.3	0.00056234	65.0
70.0	0.00031633	1.00032	1.000000	0.99968	3,162.3	0.00031623	1.00063	0.99937	10^7	3,162.3	0.00031623	70.0
75.0	0.00017786	1.00018	1.000000	0.99982	5,623.4	0.00017783	1.00036	0.99964	3.1623×10^7	5,623.4	0.00017783	75.0
80.0	0.00010001	1.00010	1.000000	0.99990	10,000.	0.00010000	1.00020	0.99980	10^8	10,000.	0.00010000	80.0
85.0	0.000056237	1.00006	1.000000	0.99994	17,783.	0.000056234	1.00011	0.99989	3.1623×10^8	17,783.	0.000056234	85.0
90.0	0.000031624	1.00003	1.000000	0.99997	31,623.	0.000031623	1.00006	0.99994	10^9	31,623.	0.000031623	90.0
95.0	0.000017783	1.00002	1.000000	0.99998	56,234.	0.000017783	1.00004	0.99996	3.1623×10^9	56,234.	0.000017783	95.0
100.0	0.0000100000	1.00001	1.000000	0.99999	10^5	0.000010000	1.00002	0.99998	10^{10}	10^5	0.0000100000	100.0

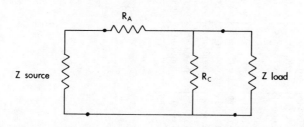

FIG. A-2.   L-pad schematic for larger source impedance than load impedance.

L-PAD ATTENUATOR

An attenuator deserving special mention is the L-pad, which comprises two resistors connected in an L-shape. It has only two elements and so cannot simultaneously satisfy all three conditions listed previously but typically is used when only two of the three conditions are critical (e.g., matching network between two impedances) and the *source impedance* is to be *matched.*

Where R_s exceeds R_L, the L-pad resembles Fig. A-2, and the equations are:

$$R_A = \frac{R_s}{\sqrt{\dfrac{R_s}{R_L}}} \left(\frac{k\sqrt{\dfrac{R_s}{R_L}} - 1}{k} \right)$$

$$R_C = \frac{R_s}{\sqrt{\dfrac{R_s}{R_L}}} \left(\frac{1}{k - \sqrt{\dfrac{R_s}{R_L}}} \right)$$

Where R_s is less than R_L, the L-network is reversed, as in Fig. A-3, and the equations are:

$$R_A = \frac{R_L}{\sqrt{\dfrac{R_L}{R_s}}} \left(k - \sqrt{\dfrac{R_L}{R_s}} \right)$$

$$R_C = \frac{R_L}{\sqrt{\dfrac{R_L}{R_s}}} \left(\frac{k}{k\sqrt{\dfrac{R_L}{R_s}} - 1} \right)$$

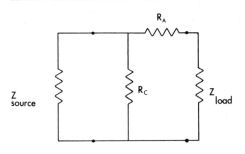

FIG. A-3.   L-pad schematic for larger load impedance than source impedance.

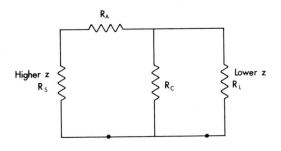

FIG. A-4.   L-pad schematic for smaller load impedance than source impedance.

If it is desired that the load impedance be matched, the networks are reversed.

An L-pad is the limiting condition of a T-pad; that is, one series arm becomes zero, and two impedances are matched with some minimal attenuation. In this instance, the series arm of the L-pad will look at the higher impedance while the parallel, or shunt, arm will connect across the lower impedance, as in Fig. A-4, and the attenuation loss can be determined by use of the equation:

$$k = \sqrt{\frac{R_s}{R_L}} + \sqrt{\frac{R_s}{R_L} - 1}$$

One solves for the values of R_A and R_C by using the equation for a T-pad attenuator having the value of k given by the equation. If a circuit requires that only one impedance be matched, the L-pad deteriorates to a single resistor. If it is desirable to terminate the larger impedance in its image impedance, the terminating resistance will be in series with the smaller impedance and will have a value of the larger impedance minus the smaller impedance. If the smaller impedance is to be matched, the larger will be shunted (paralleled) by a resistor of a size chosen to bring the combination to the value of the smaller.

BRIDGED-T ATTENUATOR NETWORK

A variety of different attenuator networks is available although none does any more than the T-pad (i.e., does any more than match source and load impedances and introduce some attenuation). The disadvantage of the T-pad is that it requires all three resistors to be variable so that exact values can be set for each. An alternative to the T-pad is a bridged-T, which requires four resistors, two of which are variable. See Fig. A-5.

For an application requiring some attenuation to isolate two circuits for which the adjacent source and load impedances are equal, the values of the resistances for a bridged-T are as follows:

$$R_s = R_L = R_B$$

$$R_A = R_B (k - 1)$$

$$R_C = R_B \left(\frac{1}{k - 1} \right)$$

PI-ATTENUATOR

One additional common and useful attenuator network for unbalanced circuitry is the pi-attenuator with a configuration as shown in Fig. A-6. The necessary equations are:

$$R_A = R_1 \frac{k^2 - 1}{k^2 - 2k \sqrt{\dfrac{R_1}{R_2} + 1}}$$

$$R_B = \sqrt{\frac{R_1 R_2}{2} - \left(\frac{k^2 - 1}{1} \right)}$$

$$R_C = R_2 \left(\frac{k^2 - 1}{k^2 - 2 \dfrac{k}{\sqrt{\dfrac{R_1}{R_2}}}} + 1 \right)$$

There are several varieties of additional unbalanced attenuator networks, but the above should suffice for most applications of interest.

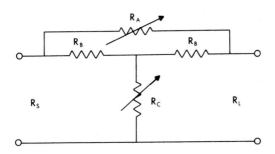

FIG. A-5.   Bridged-T schematic.

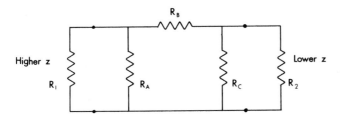

FIG. A-6.   Pi-attenuator schematic.

Balanced Network Attenuators

All of the attenuators previously discussed insert resistance into one side of the line only. For circuits in applications using balanced lines, balanced attenuators are necessary. A balanced attenuator is made by constructing two unbalanced networks, with each connected between ground or the central top point of the attenuator and one side of the line.

BALANCED T-NETWORK

For example, the balanced-T (sometimes called the balanced-H) network is as shown in Fig. A-7.

$$R_A = \frac{R_1}{2}\left(\frac{k^2 + 1}{k^2 - 1}\right) - \sqrt{R_1 R_2}\left(\frac{k}{k^2 - 1}\right)$$

$$R_B = \frac{R_2}{2}\left(\frac{k^2 + 1}{k^2 - 1}\right) - \sqrt{R_1 R_2}\left(\frac{k}{k^2 - 1}\right)$$

$$R_C = \sqrt{R_1 R_2}\left(\frac{k}{k - 1}\right)$$

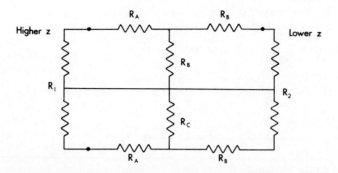

FIG. A-7.   Balanced-T (or balanced-H) pad schematic.

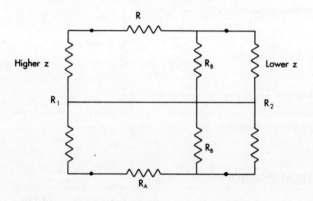

FIG. A-8.   Balanced-L (or balanced-U) pad schematic with larger source than load impedance.

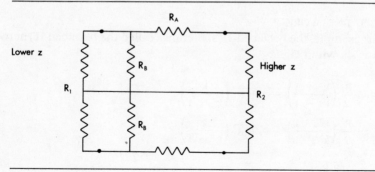

FIG. A-9.   Balanced-L (or balanced-U) pad schematic with larger load than source impedance.

The reader may note that the equations for the balanced-T yield values that are just half of those obtained for the T-pad.

BALANCED L-PAD

Creating a balanced L-pad (also called a balanced-U) involves, in like manner to the balanced-T, connecting two unbalanced L-pads, each between the center of the attenuator and one side of the line, as in Figs. A-8 and A-9.

To match the higher impedance:

$$R_A = \frac{R_1}{2\sqrt{\dfrac{R_1}{R_2}}} \left(\frac{k\sqrt{\dfrac{R_1}{R_z}} - 1}{k} \right)$$

$$R_B = \frac{R_1}{2\sqrt{\dfrac{R_1}{R_2}}} \left(\frac{1}{k - \sqrt{\dfrac{R_1}{R_z}}} \right)$$

To match the lower impedance:

$$R_A = \frac{R_2}{2\sqrt{\dfrac{R_2}{R_1}}} \left(k - \sqrt{\dfrac{R_2}{R_1}} \right)$$

$$R_B = \frac{R_2}{2\sqrt{\dfrac{R_2}{R_1}}} \left(\frac{k}{k\sqrt{\dfrac{R_2}{R_1}} - 1} \right)$$

Again, the reader may note that the equations for the balanced-L yield values just half of those obtained for the comparable L-pad.

Index

Index